Food Allergy-Facts and Principles

Dr.S. Parameshwari

Published by

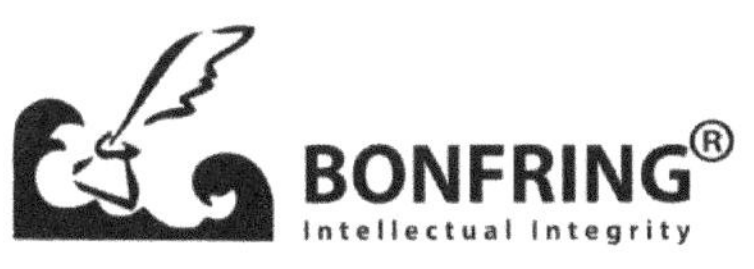

Food Allergy-Facts and Principles

ISBN 978-93-85477-96-6

Author

Dr.S. Parameshwari

Bonfring
309, 2nd Floor, 5th Street Extension, Gandhipuram,
Coimbatore-641 012.
Tamilnadu, India.
E-mail: info@bonfring.org
Website: www.bonfring.org
Phone: 0422-3928700

Dedicated to

*My Endearing Son **Mr.S.P. Poorvaj Naresh** for his Patient Understanding, Kind Heartedness, Compromising my close Association with him in Day to-Day Life right from his Childhood when i was away from family due to my occupation. Without his Psychological Emotional Cooperation i couldnot Progress.*

Preface

From My Journey of cumulative seventeen years of experience in both Teaching in STET Women's College, Mannargudi and Dietician in Tamilnadu, Govt. Medical College at Kilpauk, Chennai as Counselling Dietician, Govt Medical College Thanjavur as Administrative and Counselling Dietician, Apart from Teaching Foods, Nutrition and Dietetics to Under Graduate, Post Graduate and M.Phil., Research Scholar Students made me to felt the need for a reference book that deals in all areas of Nutrition and Dietetics in an easily understandable way for students as well for any person who is interested in nutrition. During my dedicated work experience of dietician coming across people with many illness poor knowledge about nutrition in disease conditions even among the well educated patients ,seeing the sufferings of thousands of patients in medical college wards during counselling made a strong drive which prompted me to write a book on many aspects of nutrition and dietetics. And with my sustained efforts **"FOOD ALLERGY-FACTS AND PRINCIPLES"** materialized in the form of book which is one among the book i focused. Every effort has been made to make it a useful reference book for BSc Nutrition & Dietetics and BSc Nursing students.

Prevention of food allergies can be achieved   through lifestyle modification and elimination of certain allergy producing foods. This book focuses not only on the basic facts but also reflects the ways and means we can avoid or reduce the allergic situation. The dietary management of allergy is the foremost concern and due importance is highlighted in diet areas.

This book contains thirteen chapters in a coherent manner. To start with introduction of food allergy, it describes immunological basis of allergy, common food allergens, characteristics and development of food allergy. Apart from above areas it also describes about hazards, symptoms, clinical manifestations, diagnosis and treatment of food allergy. The most important aspect of allergy viz. prevention, patient counseling and nutrition management of food allergy is very well explained.

The herculaean task of writing this book cannot be fulfilled and come into limelight in the world, unless i bow to my head to my most affectionate husband and endearing my son who had shared my sufferings and shouldered the pains during this course of book writing. My indebtedness towards my family members cannot be expressed in words. The Words ceased to mean to express my emotions and bondness on my family members especially to my son. The necessary suggestions, technical inputs, outlay about book, the clinical points inclusion and technical inputs to improve the soundness of book, inputs given by husband is highly commendable, laudable and it cannot be compared in any way.

Dr.S. Parameshwari

Acknowledgement

It is my pleasure and deep sense of indebtedness to scientists and publishers if a number of standard books and journals of Indian and Foreign origin were used.

My indebtedness and words of thankfulness goes to my husband **Dr.CS. Sakthivelan**, My Son **Mr.S.P. Poorvaj Naresh** throughout my pathway of writing this book for their sustained moral, physical and technical support in bringing this book to the world and who spared their valuable time in helping me.

It is my best way of expressing my deeply felt sense of gratitude ,appreciation and extending my warm heartfelt thanks to my sincere Research Scholars **Ms.P. Sasikala**, Assistant Professor and **Mrs.C. Roselin**, Assistant Professor, Cauvery College for Women, Trichy and **Mrs. Mathangi,** Assistant Professor, V.V.Vanniyaperumal College for Women, Virudhunagar.

I am grateful to students and faculty members of different colleges whose encouragement inspired me to bring this book.

My Soul of Inspiration and Breath of Reciprocating the Laurels of My Heights of Growth in Education is due, unless I proudly patiently acknowledge the STET WOMEN'S COLLEGE, MANNARKUDI Correspondent, Principal, Endearing N&D Department Staffs and friends of STET. It is my pleasure to specially acknowledge STET WOMEN'S COLLEGE, MANNARKUDI which shaped my carrier.

Last but not the least ,it is my maternal inclination to show my affinity and growth towards my parents that i am very much thankful and submit my humbleness to my father and my mother whose dedication made my growth in increasing all the way of my life. Growth in my carrier cannot be completed unless i thank my emotionally bind brother and his family.

I also thank the **Bonfring Publication** for bringing out this book in a nice way.

Above all

I SING GLORY TO ALMIGHTY GOD FOR GIVING ME GOOD HEALTH, SOUL AND SUSTAINED BLESSINGS IN ALL MY ENDEAVOURS.

Author Profile

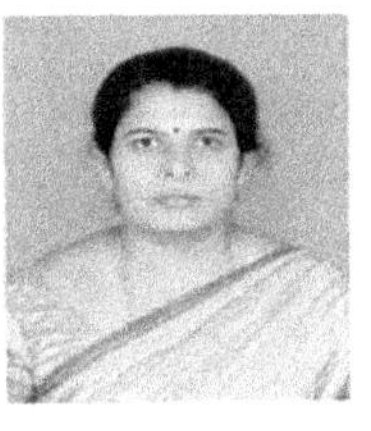

Dr.S. Parameshwari

Assistant Professor

Dept. of Home Science

Mother Teresa Women's University

Kodaikanal

Dr.S. Parameshwari MSc., MPhil., PhD., is currently working as Assistant Professor, Dept. of Home Science, Mother Teresa Women's University, Kodaikanal. She had an experience of 10 years as LECTURER AND HEAD in the Dept. of NUTRITION AND DIETETICS, STET WOMEN's COLLEGE, MANNARKUDI.

She served as a Board of studies Member in Home Science(UG), Nutrition and Dietetics(PG), Bharathidasan University, Tiruchirapalli for Three Years. Then she joined Tamil Nadu Health Department as DIETICIAN in Govt. Medical College Kilpauk, Chennai and later in Thanjavur Medical College.

During her tenure as Dietician, she implemented New Diet Pattern in Thanjavur Medical College. She documented so many Diet Awareness Programmes like World Diabetes Day and various ICT Material for Diet Counselling for Communicable and Non communicable Diseases. During her Dietician Period, she conducted various pilot studies on Diet Supplementation, Fortification Studies, Food Consumption Patterns, Clinical Surveys and conducted several Diet trial Studies. She participated Tamil Nadu Govt Noon Meal Scheme Evaluation Studies in Salem District conducted by Salem District Administration. She had counselling experience of more than three thousand patients with multiple diseases including cancer patients and revival of burn injury patients.

Then She joined as Assistant Professor in the Dept. of Home Science, Mother Teresa Women's University, Kodaikanal. She Guided more than 15 MPhil. Research Scholars. She published more than 15 Research Papers in Reputed National and International Journals. She served as an invited speaker in various colleges as resource person. She Participated more than 25 National, International Conferences and Seminars and Presented her Papers. She is member of more than 6 Professional Bodies. She published few books in Foods and Nutrition.

<table>
<tr><th>Chapter</th><th>Contents</th><th>Page No</th></tr>
</table>

CHAPTER I

INTRODUCTION

Allergy is one of the medical distress due to food is a concern for mankind nowadays. An allergic reaction is really an immune reaction. It is reaction against foreign intrusion by the body's defensive mechanisms, the antibodies. The body manufactures different groups of antibodies, or Immunoglobulins as they are called, and the one we are concerned with, in allergy is Immunoglobulin-E (IgE).

Everyone produces some IgE as an immune response, but allergic persons produce a greater quantity of IgE.

Allergy is an abnormal reaction of the body's antibody antigen defense mechanism. There appears to be an excessive production of immunoglobulin E(IgE), which in turn over reacts with the allergen (antigen) to produce the symptoms. An allergen is the substance that sets off the reaction. In most instances the allergen is protein in nature, but non protein substances such as aspirin can also cause reactions.

IgE antibodies are bound to special white blood cells and to mast cell in the tissues, particularly in the so-called shock organs of the body- the smooth muscles, mucous glands, mucous membranes and the skin. When allergens arrive on the scene, allergens and antibodies battle starts. In the process, the body suffers damages, either directly or indirectly, because during the struggle chemical mediators such as histamines are released. Normally bound to mast cells and inactive, these substances once released, may be none food friendly to their host. They are thought to be responsible for the immediate reaction in the shock organs with symptoms of hives, swollen nasal membranes, wheezing, and the like.

i. Nature of Food Allergy

A problem specific to childhood but occurring at all ages through the life cycle is that of food allergy. Because of the possible effect of food allergy on nutrient utilization and the stress on the body imposed by the allergy, individuals are placed at nutritional risk, with the growth and development of children particularly threatened. Good management is imperative and includes Strict Avoidance of the Offending Foods and Awareness of the Age–Specific Nutritional Needs.

First Factor: Actually, probably the most important reason some people become allergic and others do not, is most probably due to a hereditary factor. In some families allergy runs strong and those born into these families may inherit the tendency. Studies have shown that an individual has nearly a 75 percent chance of being allergic if both his/her parents have allergies. He is also likely to develop his own brand of allergy at an earlier age. If one parent is allergic or allergy runs in one side of the family, the child has close to a 50 percent chance of developing allergy.

A Second Factor in the development of allergy disease is the duration and amount of exposure to allergens the individual suffers.

A Third Factor is the nature of the allergen itself. Some are more potent than others. Among inhalants, ragweed pollen is more potent than grass pollen. Among foods, citrus fruits are more potent allergens than apples, pears than carrots, cow's milk than soybean milk.

A Fourth Factor is the individual's physical condition at the time of exposure to an allergen. If he has a cold, ragweed pollen may cause an allergic reaction that he would not have suffered otherwise. If he has a stomach already upset by infection or is suffering from diarrhea, more food allergens may be absorbed into his blood stream and will intensify his symptoms of allergic reaction. Infection seems to lower a person's tolerance to some allergens.

A Fifth Factor and perhaps the strongest of all is the role of emotions in allergy. Emotional stress may precipitate allergy and greatly aggravate its symptoms. Some allergists insist that emotions trigger but not to cause allergy–that an underlying allergy was already present. Others state that the effect of the emotions on the allergy is to cause leakage of fluid from the blood vessels, producing an allergic condition.

There are other factors that play a lesser role in allergy. Weather and the Seasons, for instance, have an effect on our ability to react normally or abnormally to various allergens. Sudden changes of temperature may trigger an existing allergy, especially Asthma. The relationship of climate and geographic location to food allergy is not clear, but these factors play a larger role in other allergies, particularly in inhalant allergy caused by pollens, house dust and mold.

There is also the possibility that various aspects of bodily makeup and metabolism have something to do with allergic sensitivity. Hyperthyroid conditions may be conducive to allergy, perhaps because the person with an overactive thyroid gland reacts with excessive sensitivity to a number of external irritants.

Certain types of skin such as those incapable of neutralizing alkali substances efficiently, tend to have contact dermatitis (inflammation of the skin). People with such skin have greater difficulty with all sorts of materials including soap.

Allergy can appear at any age, but about half of the adult allergies begin in childhood usually before puberty. Even if the symptoms disappear, these childhood allergies really are not out grown. The tendency is still there and allergy may surface again, in the same form or in other forms later in life. This is especially true if childhood allergies have gone untreated and uncontrolled. Earlier the allergy is diagnosed and managed, the better the chances it can be controlled and the lesser the chances of developing new allergies in later life. An unrecognized and untreated childhood allergy may come back to a plague, in person of his/her forty age.

As a person's sensitivity becomes more severe, the number of substances he reacts to become more numerous.

Allergies are initiated in four ways:

1. *by contact with foods, drugs, aerosol sprays, pesticides, poison ivy, hair, molds*
2. *by ingestion of foods, drugs*
3. *by inhalation of pollens, dust, cosmetics, sprays, molds, perfumes*
4. *by injection of vaccines, serum, hormones, antibiotics, insect bites*

ii. Definition

Terms commonly used to describe an adverse reaction to foods include Food Allergy, Hypersensitivity, Sensitivity, and Intolerance. Strictly speaking, these terms are not synonymous.

Food Allergy or Hypersensitivity denotes an adverse immunologic response to a substance with characteristic symptoms whenever the food is ingested.

Food Sensitivity is a slightly broader term applied to conditions in which an abnormal reaction occurs following ingestion of specific foods and in which an immunologic etiology is likely, but not proven.

Food Intolerance, on the other hand, does not involve an immunologic mechanism and may be due to an enzyme deficiency or other factors.

In Food Allergy, symptoms are produced within minutes or a few hours following ingestion of the food and the reaction occurs whenever the food is ingested.

In Food Sensitivity or Intolerance symptoms may occur hours or days after ingestion of the food substance and the condition tends to improve spontaneously or following a period of elimination of the food.

Allergen/Antigen

The substances responsible for initiation of the allergic reaction are called Allergen or Antigen. It is usually a protein, but may be a polysaccharide, or a substance that binds to a protein to form a complex which becomes the active allergen.

Allergy may be defined as an adverse immunological reaction to a substance that is harmless in similar amounts to the majority of people.

Food allergy or a reaction to food, can affect the gastrointestinal tract, in which case it is called a gastro intestinal allergy or it can affect any other body system. Food allergy is an immune reaction and must be differentiated from food intolerance, which may be due to an enzyme deficiency, digestive problem or psychological reaction.

CHAPTER II

IMMUNOLOGICAL BASIS OF ALLERGY

An allergy is the abnormal reaction or hypersensitivity to a substance which produces symptoms in the allergic individual. Although the allergy can appear at any age, it is far more common in infants and children. It has been estimated that approximately half of adult allergies begin in childhood. The sensitivity to a particular food may seem to disappear with increasing age, but the tendency is never completely outgrown.

In the case of food allergy, the antigens are natural products, usually protein that are ingested in food. Since the body regards these as intruding substances, it produces an antibody which binds the antigen. Antibodies also known as immunoglobulins, are found in the blood or tissue of all healthy persons. However the allergic individual produces a greater quantity than normal, particularly immunoglobulin IgE, which creates an overreaction of this protective mechanism.

IgE is present in high concentration in the mucosa of the gastrointestinal tract, bronchial tubes and nose. These are referred to as the allergy "Shock Organs" and are very frequently the sites for the antigen antibody reactions of food allergy.

During the process of digestion, most food antigens are destroyed by the gastrointestinal tract. Because the protein molecules are very large they rarely enter the bloodstream. The higher incidence of food allergy in infants and young children is thought to be related to the lower efficiency of their immature gastro intestinal food and consequently more antigens of food allergens to be absorbed into the blood stream for reaction with antibodies complex which becomes the active allergen.

In most individuals, food antigens are destroyed in the gastrointestinal tract; however, in atopic persons, those with a predisposition to allergy, after repeated exposure to the allergen, the antigen is absorbed from the gastrointestinal tract and enters the circulation. In infants and young children food allergy is usually attributed to an immature gastrointestinal tract which permits passage of the   antigenically active substance into the circulation.

Immune System

The immune system function is to clear the body of foreign substances (or antigens), such as viruses, bacteria, blood cells and tissue cells. Normally when antigens interact with cells of the immune system they are cleared from the body without any adverse reaction. Three type of cells respond to antigens presented; B lymphocytes, T lymphocytes, and Macrophages. The lymphocytes arise from stem cells in the bone marrow and along with T cells originating from stem cells in the Thymus, are the basis for the function of the two branches of the immune system; the Humoral Pathway and the Cell Mediated Pathway.

Humoral Immunity (Humoral Pathway)

It involves Antibodies (Immunoglobulins) which play an important role in food allergy. Antigen – specific antibodies are produced by the B lymphocytes (B cells) in response to the antigen presented. The union of an antigen and its antibody results in the production of chemical mediators or direct cellular damage, which in turn causes symptoms.

Five Classes of Antibodies have been identified.

1. *IgG, IgM, and IgD Antibodies protect the body against bacteria and viruses. Secretory IgA antibodies-present in breast milk provides breast-feeding infants with local intestinal protection against viruses and bacteria.*

2. *IgA antibodies: Present in saliva and intestinal secretions block the absorption of antigens.*

3. *IgE antibodies help to eliminate parasites from the body, and are also responsible for classic allergic reactions.*

Cellular or Cell-Mediated Immunity

It involves the action of T lymphocytes (T cells). T cells do not produce antibodies, but do recognize antigens. When antigens stimulate T-cell growth, the T cell produce lymphokines and cytokines, substances that help to regulate the activities of other cells or that cause direct cellular damage to target cells, resulting in the destruction of antigens. Cellular Immunity has an important role in resistance to viruses, fungi, tumor cells, and other foreign cells. Certain reactions, contact dermatitis and the tuberculin reactions are also mediated by T cells. The role of Cellular Immunity in food allergy is unclear.

Tissue Macrophages derived from Monocytes present in the blood also have an important role in the blood, also have important roles in the recognition and clearance of antigens. Through the process of Phagocytosis, the Macrophage engulfs and destroys Antigens. B cells, T cells and Macrophages are all thought to interact.

The Thymus and Tonsils also play a role in immunity. The Thymus is a Ductless Gland like organ which produces T-cell, is essential to the development of Peripheral Lymphoid Tissue. Although the Thymus is the largest and most active prior to puberty, the mature T cells that it exports, exert their effect in adulthood. Removal of the Thymus during adulthood has little effect on a person's resistance to disease.

The Tonsils consist of two small, rounded masses of lymphoid tissue that is present in the path of inspired air and all ingested food and liquids. Foreign material that is inspired into the airways and that becomes trapped in the tonsillar crypts comes in contact with antigen processing cells. Their surgical removal, especially during childhood may impair or delay the development of an individual's immunity to disease.

Types of Allergic Reaction*

Reaction/Classification	Mechanism	Comments
Type 1 Immediate Hypersensitivity, Anaphylactic IgE-Mediated, or reagenic Reaction	Allergen binds with sensitized IgE antibody on mast cell (specialized granular cells in the intestines, skin, and respiratory tract) or basophils (similar cells in blood). This results in release of mediators (histamine eosinophilic chemotactic factor, bradykinin, and so forth). IgG has also been identified as being involved in this type of reaction.	Includes hay fever, anaphylaxis, most food allergies. Symptoms occur within seconds or up to 2 hours. Symptoms of food reactions may include laryngeal edema, vomiting, diarrhea, eczema, itching, bronchospasm, and shock.
Type 2 Cytotoxic	IgG antibody reacts with cell membrane or antigen associated with cell membrane.	Results from transfusion of in compatible blood types. No food reactions have been demonstrated
Type 3 Antigen-antibody complex Arthusreacton	Antigen and antibodies (IgG and IgM) form a complex called "precipitating antibody". The antigen antibody complex is and an Arthus reaction when it occurs in soft tissues like blood vessels, lungs, or kidneys, and is serum sickness when the complex circulates. Activation of complement also occurs in some cases.	Occurs in some food reactions; milk precipitins have been found in lungs of some children with chronic respiratory infection, and in GI tract in those with gastroenteropathies. Reactions usually take 6 hours or more to appear and may take several days to be clinically apparent.
Type 4 Delayed or cell mediated hypersensitivity	T cells interact directly with antigen.	Usual mechanism of graft rejection. Possibly involved in some food allergies, such as protein-losing enteropathies and celiac disease.]

*Adopted from Butkus SN and Mahan LK: Food allergies: Immunoloical reactions to foods. The American Dietetic Association. Reprinted by permission from journal of the American Dietetic Association, vol 86, p 601,1986.

Immunologic Basis: Antigen Exclusion

In order for an allergic reaction to a food to occur, proteins or other large molecules from the food (antigens/allergens) must be absorbed from the gastrointestinal tract, interact with the immune system and produce a response. Under normal conditions, the gastrointestinal tract and the immune system provide a barrier that prevents the absorption of most intact proteins. When this barrier fails, allergic sensitization may occur and re-exposure produces an allergic reaction. Some simple chemical substances (small molecules) can become allergens by combining with larger proteins.

Relationship of Immunological Factors to Symptoms or Signs

Antibodies	Symptoms or Signs	Timing
IgE	Rhinitis,Asthma, Urticaria, Abdominal pain, "Rash"	Immediate (Minutes)
IgG, IgM	Urticaria, Inflammation, Edema, Eczema, Asthma	Early (Hours)
IgA	Malabsorption, Enteropathy	
IgG, IgM	Nephritis, Arthritis, Fever "Rash"	Late (Weeks)
Cellular	Unknown Effects	

CHAPTER III

COMMON FOOD ALLERGENS

Many foods have been implicated in food allergy. However relatively few foods have been documented to cause adverse reactions. The most common food allergens are commonly eaten foods with high-protein content, especially of Plant or Marine origin (Taylor et al, 1987). In Children the foods most commonly documented to cause reactions are Cow's Milk, Soy, Peanut, Egg, Wheat and Fish (Bock, 1987; Eggleston, 1987; Marshall et al, 1984; Sampson, 1988). However, food allergy may develop to any food included in the Diet (Bock, 1987). Positive reactions following ingestion of corn, rice, rye, nuts, shrimp, chicken, turkey, pork, beef, bananas, squash, and potatoes have also been reported (Bock, 1986 and 1987; Sampson, 1988). Reactions to shellfish, peanuts, nuts, and grains have been described in the adult population (Atkins et al, 1985; Bernstein at al 1982).

The antigens in food are often large proteins (M Wt.- 10,000 to 70,000 Daltons). Individual foods contain many different proteins, of which only a few may be highly allergenic. For example, cow's milk contains more than 20 different proteins, of which beta–lacto globulin, casein, and alphalactalbumin are among the most allergenic. Cross reactivity between antigens may occur especially between foods within the same biologic family. For example, an infant who is allergic to cow's milk may be allergic to goat's milk. A child who is allergic to ragweed pollen may not tolerate watermelon. However, allergy to one food or pollen does not necessarily mean that there will be an allergy to all related foods. In children, clinically significant cross reactivity between legumes, such as peanut and soybean is rare (Berhisel – Broadbent and Sampson, 1989). Adverse reactions to each food must be documented.

Although many allergens are unaffected by denaturation caused by heat and acid, the allergenicity of some proteins can be altered by heating (Aas, 1984). Antigens of some foods are removed by processing. For example, individuals sensitive to soybeans, cottonseed, peanuts, or corn usually tolerate soy, cottonseed, peanut, or corn oil, respectively (American Academy of Allergy and Immunology, 1984; Bush et al, 1984, Taylor et al, 1981 and 1985). However, caution is advised for those with a history of severe anaphylactic reactions (American Academy of Allergy and Immunology(1984).

Food Allergens

Any food may produce reactions, but the most frequent offenders are milk, eggs, wheat, citrus fruits, chocolate or cola, legumes, nuts, tomatoes, corn, fish, shellfish and some spices. It is the protein component of the foods which is considered to be the cause of allergy. The increasing incidence of food allergies due to use of soy products and food additives are of some concern.

Foods unlike in flavor and structure but belonging to the same botanic group may result in allergic manifestations. For example, buckwheat is not of the cereal family but in a group that includes rhubarb. The sweet potato is not related to the white potato but is a member of the morning glory family. Spinach, a frequent reactor, is in the same family with beets. The following botanic classification of a few common foods illustrates the relationship of foods that at first appear to be dissimilar.

- **Cereal:** wheat, rye, barely, rice, oats, malt, corn sorghum, cane sugar.
- **Lily:** onion, garlic, asparagus, chives, leeks, shallots
- **Gourd:** squash, pumpkin, cucumber, cantaloups watermelon.
- **Cabbage and mustard:** turnips cabbage, collards, cauliflower, broccoli, kale, radish, horseradish, watercress, Brussels sprouts.

Common Food Allergies

A person may become allergic to a food or other allergen at any age, but usually begins to have symptoms in childhood. A very early allergic reaction (in the first five days of life) means that the neonate was probably sensitized in -utero, because of the mother's overindulgence in allergenic foods such as eggs or milk. The sensitivity may wear off, or the person may become desensitized and entirely free from the disturbance that affected him in childhood. Foods that belong to the same botanical group may produce a similar allergic reaction, for example, cabbage and cauliflower or orange and grapefruit. Furthermore, an allergic individual who experiences a reaction to a given food may on another day eat the same food without reaction. This may be due to his general physical condition and the complexity of immune reactions. An allergic response may occur only when the individual is fatigued or emotionally upset.

Protein

Any food can produce allergic manifestations. However, it is believed that protein is the important factor in food allergy, although the offending food may contain only a minute amount of it. Among the most common offenders are wheat, milk, eggs, fish, shellfish, strawberries, tomatoes and chocolate. Others to be considered are pork, oranges, spices, condiments, nuts, corn, asparagus, spinach, cabbage, celery, onion, garlic and rhubarb. The ingestion of the smallest quantity of an offending food may produce symptoms or reaction. Therefore, it is necessary for the allergic individual to analyze the prepared foods and food combinations before eating them. For example, sausage may contain wheat and the small amount of wheat could cause an allergic disturbance.

Milk Allergy

Milk Allergy is usually thought to be the most common allergy in infants and young children. The estimated frequency of occurrence in children ranges from 0.3 to 7 percent, with the onset most commonly prior to 1 month of age. Part of the reason that milk is such a frequent offender is its high level of consumption particularly in infancy. The sensitivity may be due to one of three proteins found in milk; lactolbumin, lactoglobulin and casein. Lactalbumin plays the primary role in allergic reactions. Symptoms often related to milk allergy are eczema, colic, mucous and bloody diarrhea and asthma.

Iron deficiency anemia and intestinal loss of blood and protein have been noted to result from high intakes of pasteurized cow's milk. These conditions occur primarily in babies under 1 year of age whose milk intake is over 1 liter per day. Heat treatment of commercially prepared formulas seems to alleviate this problem, thus making heat liable milk protein the suspected cause of the infant's difficulty.

Wheat Allergy

There are many proteins in wheat that may act as antigens. These allergens are responsible for celiac disease, the intestinal malabsorption condition that occurs in children. Antibodies are produced in the intestinal mucosa and form an immune reaction following ingestion of wheat. The antigen–antibody complex injures the mucosa, resulting in loss of protein from the gut. Wheat allergy is the most common cereal allergy but many children are also sensitive to corn. *Rice is the grain that is least likely to produce an allergic manifestation.*

Egg Allergy

Egg is an important allergen, frequently causing violent and almost instantaneous reactions, Egg, allergy, often manifesting as eczema or urticaria is most common in infancy and early childhood. The sensitivity is in response to the albumin, the protein in the egg white and may even be induced by inhaling the odour of cooking eggs. Although it is not as commonly a problem as the albumin of the egg white, the egg yolk can also cause symptoms. Because many vaccines are often grown on egg or chick embryo, the egg-sensitive child must be guarded against such inoculations, which may have dangerous effects.

Other Allergens in Food

A food contaminant such as trace amounts of penicillin in cow's milk may also be an allergen. An allergen may be one of the many substances added to processed foods. These substances such as Artificial colours, Artificial flavours, Spices and other food additives should always be tested for in cases of unexplained allergy. The fruits most commonly producing an allergy in children are citrus fruits, strawberries, and melons. Group allergies may occur among fruits. For example, a child who is allergic to oranges may often be sensitive to other citrus fruits–lemon, grapefruit, and lime. Urticaria seems to be a symptom often associated with fruit allergies. Of the vegetables, tomatoes and the legumes, (including peanuts) are the most common offenders.

Fish and Seafood are also potent allergens. Some children are sensitive to fish but can tolerate shellfish, whereas others have a generalized allergy to all types of seafood. Symptoms often reported from fish allergy include urticaria, gastrointestinal problems, and migraine headaches. Beef, pork, and poultry may cause cutaneous and respiratory problems. *Of all the meats, lamb is the least common offender.* Nuts, chocolate and cocoa, mustard, black pepper, cloves, and food additives are other reported sources of food allergy.

Food History

A carefully detailed food history should be taken for every individual suspected of having an allergy. The food history often discloses specific food allergies through the listing of disliked foods or foods that disagree with the patient. In addition, the patients should be asked about their cigarette smoking and use of aspirin antacids, chewing gum, lozenges and laxatives, which may contains substances that cause an allergic reaction.

Food Diary: If a Patient keeps a Food Diary and records the foods eaten preceding the appearance of allergic symptoms, the data will be useful for diagnosis.

Chapter IV

Characteristics of Food Allergy

The mechanism of food allergy is thought to work mainly in two ways:

1. By direct contact of food allergens with IgE antibodies in the gastro intestinal system, resulting in very swift reactions; or
2. By the absorption of allergens from the gastro intestinal tract into the blood stream, resulting in reactions in the blood or the shock organs – the smooth muscles, mucous glands and membranes and the skin.

Two important factors play a role in whether or not, sensitization takes place:

1. The condition or efficiency of the gastrointestinal tract itself
2. The nature and amount of the allergenic food consumed.

Food allergies can also affect other body systems. An allergic person can react to the smell of food. In this case, his respiratory system is the seat of sensitization, as it is in inhalant allergies. Reaction to foods inhaled is far less common than reaction to foods ingested. Some hypersensitive folk even break out in contact dermatitis, an allergic skin condition, when they handle some foods. In this case the skin is the seat of sensitization.

Any food may be the cause of allergic reactions, but the following foods are more potent allergens than other foods.

Milk	**Fish and Shellfish**
Eggs	**Berries**
Wheat	**Peas**
Chocolate	**Citrus Fruits**
Nuts	**Corn**

Perhaps it is no coincidence that all these foods are considered particularly delicious and highly nutritious.

Reasons Why Allergens may Contaminate a Food

- Common serving utensils used to serve different foods.
- Manufacture of two different food products using the same equipment, but without proper cleaning in between.
- Misleading labels (e.g. non dairy creamers that contain sodium caseinate)
- Ingredients, added for a specific purpose, are listed on the label only in general terms of their purpose, rather than as a specific ingredient (e.g. egg white that is simply listed as an emulsifier)

- Addition of an allergenic product to a second product that bears a label listing only the ingredients of the second product (e.g., mayonnaise)
- Switching of ingredients by food manufacturers (e.g. a shortage of one vegetable oil prompting substitution with another)
- An ingredient that is present in a food, but in such a low percentage that it does not have to be listed on a label. (Adapted from Steinman HA Hidden allergens in foods J Allergy ClinImmunol 98:241 1996).

1. Age at Onset of Food Allergy

Like other allergies, food hypersensitivity can come upon us at any time of life and continue to any age. It is however most common in infancy and early childhood, perhaps because the gastro intestinal system of the young are less efficient than those of their elders. Thus, more allergens may find their way into youthful blood streams to cause allergy problems. It can be said that most food allergy occurs during the first two years of life and is often replaced by allergy to inhalants. So it is obvious that cow's milk is the chief villain in an infant allergy. It is after all, the main food for the first few months.

The milk is most always a wholesome food guaranteed to make us big and strong may come as something of a shock. Milk too can, in fact cause some pretty unpleasant diseases. Recent studies in Iron Deficiency Anemia, for instance, have indicted allergy to milk as a possible cause. The Anemia is a secondary result of continuing diarrhea and loss of blood in the stools. Recurrent attacks of bronchitis have also often been traced to allergy to milk.

2. Symptoms of Food Allergy

Allergic reactions to foods can take place in almost any body system–gastrointestinal, respiratory, cutaneous(skin), urinary, nervous, mucous glands and membranes.

Gastrointestinal disorders are the most common manifestation of sensitivity to food. Food allergy symptoms may be localized in one area, such as eczema on the cheek or hands, or they may be diffuse and generalized such as eczema on the cheek or hands; or they may be diffuse and generalized such as headache, abdominal pain or behavior disorders. They may begin especially if the skin is involved at one site and gradually spread. Thus, eczema brought on by sensitivity to eggs may begin as a small patch and spread until the child or adult is covered. Symptoms of food allergy can be so varied and differ so in severity that diagnosis is a real puzzle. Not only do symptoms to a given allergen differ among patients, but they may vary in the same patient. Thus, one person may register his sensitivity to milk with diarrhea, while another will react to milk with headaches.

3. *Fixed Type of Allergic Response*

This is a designation used by some allergists to describe the sensitivity of a person who reacts to a small amount of a food at every exposure, no matter what the interval, with specific and unvarying symptoms. It is fortunately, a less common sensitivity, for the reaction is usually the most severe type producing immediate symptoms–often asthma or hives or shock. Such a patient does not develop a tolerance to the allergenic food or foods. He is usually struck with his sensitivity for life and has no other recourse than to avoid the foods that make him ill. Sometimes his sensitivity is so great that he reacts to a very small amount of the food, virtually a crumb. Sometimes these severely sensitive people need only smell or touch the food to react. Avoidance must then include such things as handing the food or being in the same area where it is being cooked. Peeling apples or slicing them might be too much for someone severely sensitive to them. If it is eggs that are an individual's undoing, he might not be able to crack them or even touch the shells. Some doctors have estimated that 5 to 10 percent of food-sensitive persons fall into the category of fixed allergic response to food.

4. *Variable or Cyclical Type of Allergic Response*

These designations or similar ones are sometimes used to indicate a sensitivity that varies not only in the amount of food needed to cause symptoms but also in the interval between ingestion and the appearance of symptoms. It is by far the most common type of allergic response to food and is much more difficult to diagnose that the fixed type of response since cause and effect fluctuate so. He can often develop tolerance to the foods causing his problems by eating less of them less frequently. If he is to remain symptoms free, though he will need to pay close attention to a number of factors that may influence this type of allergic response.

- Infection
- Stress
- Fatigue
- Overeating at one sitting
- Too frequent consumption of a specific food
- Condition of food (cooked or raw, fresh or stale)
- Presence of pollen and other allergens, such as house dust or mold
- Pollution
- Changes of temperature, especially when it drops.

5. *Allergy Load Level, or Threshold Tolerance*

Sensitivity to food may be the sole cause for symptoms, but this is less common than sensitivity to several allergens. We have noted that in a fixed type of food allergy, the sufferer reacts to a given allergen and a given amount of that allergen but that in a variable type of food allergy, other conditions or factors may play a part. Thus some allergic persons react to milk at any time, others react only during pollen season. The rest of the year they may be able to drink milk with relish. In this case sensitivity to pollen plus an underlying sensitivity to milk equals symptoms, whereas either sensitivity alone is not strong enough to produce a problem or an individual may tolerate, without symptoms, several foods when eaten separately. But, if eaten together at the same meal or combined (say, in a casserole), they may bring on a reaction. In this case the person has a mild sensitivity to each of the several foods that is not strong enough to cause symptoms when the foods are eaten separately.If however he eats them all the same time the combination of allergens tips the scale and creates reaction.

The patient's threshold of tolerance to allergens, or allergic load level, makes diagnosis difficult and treatment complex. The patient's ability to tolerate allergens, whether ingested, inhaled or absorbed (his threshold) is balanced on one end of the allergy seesaw, with allergenic substances (pollen, house dust, animal dander, mild, one or more foods) plus circumstances that lower the patient's threshold (infection, stress, fatigue) teetering on the other end. If the patient's tolerance threshold is greater than the load of allergy, he will be symptom free; but if the pressure of allergy is more than the his tolerance threshold, symptom will appear.

6. *Compounding Food Allergy*

Fatigue and Emotional Stress may also unbalance the allergy lowering a person's tolerance to a food allergen. It is well known that these two factors can lower the body's resistance. The relationship of fatigue and emotional stress to allergy is not clear-cut or simple to demonstrate. But, since flare ups allergy symptoms especially asthma and hives commonly follows. Physical and mental exhaustion and/or emotional stress, the possibility is very strong that these two factors play much the same role in susceptibility to allergy that they do in susceptibility to infection.

Changes in temperature, especially chilling, can upset the balance of some allergic persons. An individual may find for instance, that foods he ate happily all in summer no longer can be tolerated once cold weather sets in. Man has long recognized seasonal influence upon his physical and mental well-being. Spring and Fall are times of generally lowered resistance to disease and infection, which may in turn affect sensitivity to food. Given that the bodily processes fluctuate to adapt to changing environmental conditions, it does not seem odd that the individual's threshold level might also rise or fall in response to such environmental conditions.

The mother may be overindulge without developing any symptoms of allergy herself, but her overconsumption of such things as eggs and milk and wheat may ensure that her baby will suffer allergic symptoms as soon as he meets these foods.

Fetal Hiccoughs, so often a matter of paternal wonder and laughter are thought to be a response to foreign protein passed from the mother's blood stream through the placenta into the blood stream of the fetus. The nursing mother also needs to exercise moderation for she may pass on allergens to the infant through her milk, thus sensitizing him.

However the breast fed baby is seven times less likely to develop allergy than his bottle fed brother. Nevertheless, the nursing mother must dine with care, lest she expose the infant to food allergens. The infant is particularly susceptible to sensitization since his immature gastrointestinal system is often inefficient and apt to allow passage of allergens into his blood stream. And this may be the beginning of the allergen–antibody battle.

A good many factors can bounce the allergic patient up and down on that seesaw. His doctor must take his allergic load level into account, if treatment is to be successful. It is often necessary to remove more than one component of the lead if the patient is to lose his symptoms. A person suffering from a cold may suddenly find that he cannot tolerate eggs even though he was accustomed to eating them almost every morning for breakfast. Mothers often refrain from giving small children milk when they have a cold but the infection has so strained her threshold as to superimpose allergic rhinitis upon her cold symptoms. Underlying sensitivity to milk plus infection tips the child's allergy seesaw out of balance

The relationship of food allergy to other allergies, such as inhalant or drug allergies is complex. Allergy to foods may be the sole cause for allergic symptoms, or allergy to foods in conjunction with another allergy may bring on symptoms in the same patient. Thus, allergy to foods may be responsible for allergic rhinitis symptoms (cough, stuffy nose, postnasal drip) in itself. Or the food allergy may share responsibility for such symptoms with an allergy to pollen. Or food allergy may cause gastrointestinal symptoms in the patient and the allergy to pollen be solely responsible for the rhinitis symptoms.

7. *Onset and Duration of Symptoms*

Onset of symptom may occur within minutes of consumption of the allergenic food. This is especially true when the victim is severely for several hours, normally anywhere from two to ten. And sometimes a person must eat the food two or three days running before any reaction is stirred up.

Duration of symptoms and, to some extent, the degree of distress depend upon how long the allergenic food remains in the body. Complete digestion and elimination usually requires a day or so or longer, if constipation is a problem. Duration of symptoms also depends upon how quickly antibodies in shock organs and the blood unite with the invading allergens and how quickly they are exhausted. The abundance or lack of abundance of Age antibodies may also be a factor. In general, symptoms from a single ingestion of a food allergen persist at least for several hours and commonly from one to seven days. As the food allergen leaves the body and the antibodies are depleted and exhausted, symptom disappear.

Sometimes after a reaction, especially if it is severe, no symptoms will be provided for one or more weeks even if the allergenic food is eaten again. This seems to be because the antibody defenses may be worn out in need of rebuilding. It's a bit like the lull between battles when armies pull back to regroup and replenish their spent forces. This theory of a brief "refractory" period explains the recurrent nature of perennial food allergy and it is this chronic reaction to foods eaten daily that presents the most persistent symptoms.

These are the main characteristics of allergy to food. The reader may find some of them rather mysterious. Perhaps he will be comforted to know that allergists are often mystified too. It is also well to remember that much about the nature and extent of allergy to food is exceedingly controversial.

CHAPTER V

RISK FACTORS FOR THE DEVELOPMENT OF FOOD ALLERGY

The risk of developing food allergy depends on heredity, exposure to a food (antigen), gastro intestinal permeability and environmental factors. Heredity is thought to play a major role in the development of allergy. Atopy, the tendency to develop IgE mediated reactions, appears to be family and child's risk of being a topic is estimated to be 100% when both parents are atopic and only when neither parent is atopic (Ziegler et al.,)

Exposure to an antigen is a prerequisite for the development of food allergy. After the initial exposure to an antigen and sensitization of the immune allergic reactions may occur. Infants may be sensitized to an antigen in breast milk, in the case allergic reactions may occur the first when infant eats the antigen in food (Anderson) depends on gastro intestinal permeability which allows anti-penetration. Gastro intestinal permeability is thought to be greatest in early infancy and to decline with intestinal maturation as the age advances. Other conditions such as gastro intestinal disease, malnutrition, prematurity and immune deficiency states, mayalose be associated with increased permeability and the risk of developing food allergy .

The amount of antigen presented and environmental factors can also influence the development of food allergy. The effects of foods on another antigens may be additive. Clinical symptoms of food allergy may increase when inhalant allergies are exacerbated by seasonal or environmental changes. Common inhalant allergens include house dust, mites, feathers, animal dander, pollens, molds, and grain dust, similarly the effects of environmental cold, may enhance the clinical symptoms of food allergy.

For example, In Japan, rice is a more common allergen than it is in the United States.

CHAPTER VI

THE HAZARDS OF FOOD ALLERGY

Allergy to food can affect any system of the body–gastrointestinal, respiratory, cutaneous (skin), urinary, nervous and even cardio-vascular (heart and blood vessels). Symptoms themselves can range from so mild as to be scarcely noticeable to so severe as to result in collapse and death.

Symptoms of food allergy are also symptoms of many other disease, before a doctor can determine. If allergy to food is the problem, he must first rule out other possible diseases. For instance, the gastrointestinal and respiratory symptoms of cystic fibrosis in young children are very much akin to those of allergy to milk.

Gastrointestinal Tract

Since the gastrointestinal tract is the body system most commonly affected by sensitivity to food.

Mouth Area

Itching, burning and swelling of lips, tongue, gums and pharynx. Dermatitis of skin around the mouth.

- Chapped or inflamed lips.
- "Geographical" tongue (patcly, denuded areas)
- Inflammation of mouth, tongue and gums
- Canker sores
- Bad breath and bad taste in mouth.

Contact with allergenic food may cause rash or dermatitis of the skin around the mouth especially in young children, who quite frequently react to oranges and tomatoes in this fashion. A reaction of angioedema (giant hives) in the mouth area can result in considerable and sometimes dangerous swelling of the lips, tongue, soft palate and pharynx. Foods that cause this odd type of reaction are usually nuts, fish, eggs and fresh fruit particularly cantaloupes, grapefruit and berries. Sensitivity to food may be the major cause of canker sores in the mouths of older children and adults, although it is thought that the viruses also may be responsible. The foods that believed are a common cause of canker sores can be remembered easily because they begin with the letter "C".

- Condiments
- Chocolate
- Cola(Includes all soft drinks)
- Catsoup(includes all foods with tomatoes)
- Corn
- Chips (includes all potatoes and fried foods)
- Salad dressing.
- Flavorings in toothpastes, mouthwashes, candy and chewing gum may also be responsible.

Swift reactions in the mouth area, clearly connected to a food just eaten, not only often dissuade the allergic individual from consuming any more of the stuff, but are often very noticeable.

An odd feature of allergic reaction in the mouth is the "geographical" tongue, a strange-looking configuration of bald patches surrounded by reddish borders. It probably derives its name from its appearance, for, when in full bloom, the tongue looks vaguely like a map.

Throat Area

Mucus in throat (resulting in constant clearing and cough) difficulty in swallowing. A sense of a lump under breast bone often accompanied by pain.

One of the most potentially serious manifestations of gastrointestinal allergic reaction involves the larynx which may swell and choke off the wind pipe. This can be frightening, not to mention suffocating, but fortunately it is rare. More common symptoms are hoarseness and loss of voice. One doctor reported that the case of a woman who lost her voice for months at a time. Removal of milk, eggs and wheat from her diet restored her ability to talk normally.

Stomach Area

- Nausea
- Vomiting
- Heartburn
- Sour sensations
- Bloating
- Belching

- Spasms of the opening between stomach and duodenum (pylorus)Symptoms of the stomach are often lumped together and called nervous indigestion. Probably most of these symptoms do represent intolerance to such foods allergens. But adults may suffer stomach distress in response to eggs and milk. Foods one would never place in the same indigestible category with onions or cucumbers or radishes.

Nausea and vomiting, of course, are symptoms of many ailments. Common especially to children. They usually do not stand alone as symptoms of food allergy but are accompanied by other discomforts such as asthma. hives, headache, abdominal pain or diarrhoea. Infants vomit with discouraging frequency, but nausea and vomiting in older children may be of a cyclic type, with sudden attacks lasting a day or two and reoccurring every few weeks. Such a syndrome may go on for years and may be accompanied by severe headache or migraine. Some doctors believe food allergy makes a large contribution to this syndrome, others consider its role negligible

Intestinal Area

- Acute abdominal pain (colic in infants)
- Subacute abdominal pain
- Diarrhoea
- Constipation
- Blood in stools
- Mucous colitis

The number one symptom of gastrointestinal allergy is abdominal pain; this is true in the infant, in the older child and the adult. Much too often such pain is dismissed summarily as being emotional in origin. Not necessarily so, although emotions, tension and stress may aggravate an existing allergy. The pain can be very real and intense that it has been mistaken for appendicitis or obstruction on occasion. The sufferer has sometimes been wheeled into surgery on this basis. Acute abdominal pain is occasionally designated as "abdominal migraine" and is thought to be caused by edema (swelling) of the gastrointestinal mucous membranes, either by direct contact with a food allergen or by the allergen – antibody battle that is going on. When other allergic symptoms are present, such as nasal discomfort or hives, the doctor may suspect that allergy is the correct diagnosis, but he will have to rule out such possibilities as appendicitis, intestinal parasites, inflammation of the colon or intestines and lead poisoning. Allergic abdominal pain can be localized or diffuse. It is usually recurrent, especially in children. Thus, when a child complains that his stomach aches after polishing off a breakfast of eggs and a glass of milk, he may not just be trying to get out of going to school. He may be suffering an allergic reaction to that health breakfast he just downed. Abdominal pain in the infant commonly occurs two or three weeks after birth. One day the baby suddenly turns red in the face, pulls up his little legs and howls.

There are other good reasons for colic, but allergy to cow's milk is a major one and it is far more common a cause than many people realize. As the saying goes, cow's milk is for calves, human milk for babies. Usually, colic does not strike immediately. The exception is the infant who may already have been sensitized in his mother's womb, it is thought that such a child arrives with his allergy to milk full-blown. In general, it can be said that the later the onset of colic, the milder it will be.

Diarrhea, too can be allergic in origin, especially in infants and young children. Often as not, milk is the cause. Even soybean milk commonly used as a substitute when cow's milk gives trouble can also bring on diarrhea. There are other causes, of course parasites, growths and infections. Again, diagnosis is make easier by the presence of other allergic symptoms, but they may or may not occur. Gastrointestinal symptoms of vomiting and cramping often do accompany diarrhea, However, Foods commonly at fault seems to be fresh vegetables such as lettuce, tomatoes and spinach. The basic trio of milk, eggs and wheat are also often indicted.

Persistent constipation may be also due to food allergy.

Mucous Colitis is another symptom. Mucous Colitis is characterized by the passing of a great deal of mucus in the stools, cramping in the abdomen and diarrhea. It is also often accompanied by other signs of allergy such as hives, hay fever and asthma. Finally, rectal pain and itching in the anal area seems to be a more frequent manifestation of sensitivity to food and Black Pepper is a common cause for such symptoms in older children and adults.

Rectal Area

- Anal Itching
- Rectal Bleeding
- Inflammation of rectum and anus
- Tenusmus (persistence desire to empty bowel and straining without result)

There are several disease syndromes associated with possible foods allergy. The two most common are celiac disease, characterized by recurrent diarrhea and what seems to be an intolerance to wheat gluten and ulcerative colitis, characterized by recurrent and often bloody diarrhea. There is also a possibility that sudden crib death in infants may be due to sensitization to milk.

Allergy antibodies lie in wait in the cells of various body tissues and in special white blood cells. When the right food allergen comes along in the blood stream, the IgE antibodies pounce. The battle is on. Wherever the antibodies are clustered in quantity–lungs, skin or brain, the struggle is fierce enough to cause symptoms. And so a bit of egg can be the cause of a stuffy nose or eczema or peculiar behavior, if our blood carries allergens to those parts of the body.

Anaphylactic Shock

One of the most severe allergy manifestations fortunately rare in food allergy is anaphylactic stock. *Its symptoms commonly are the following.*

- *Widespread Hives*
- *Nausea and Vomiting*
- *Sneezing, Wheezing*
- *Signs of Weakness*
- *Complaints of Chest Constriction*
- *Breathlessness and difficulty in breathing*
- *Anxiety, Confusion and Collapse*

Medical help must be sought immediately. There is no time to lose, for death can come very quickly. Nuts, Peanuts (which belong to the legume family) and Shellfish are the foods most often indicted in anaphylactic shock.

Respiratory System

The respiratory system seems far removed from our digestive processes, too far to be affected by the foods we eat. No area of the body is too remote for food allergens. Allergy to food does play a role in Asthma, Allergic Rhinitis and Ear problems.

Asthma

This is a severe allergy symptom. For some asthmatic patients, especially children, foods are the culprits. There is no doubt that inhalant allergens play the larger role in asthma, but recurrent perennial wheezing plus a near constant cold from fall to spring may well be blamed on food allergens as well. When asthma is not relieved by removing house dust or mold or animal dander's from the environment, the possibility of food allergy must be considered.

Asthma is a debilitating disease. When the allergen–antibody struggle takes place histamine or other mediators may be released to cause the smooth muscles wrapped around the bronchi and smaller airways to constrict, narrowing air passages. At the same time, these mediators may cause the mucous membranes lining the air passages to swell, further obstructing the airways and the mucous glands to produce mucus in great quantity. The asthmatic individual finds himself struggling not only to get air into his lungs, but also to empty the stale air from his lungs. Mucous plugs formed, because of the over secretion of the glands, making the effort to expel air increasingly difficult as the intake of fresh air lessens. The characteristic wheezing of asthma is caused by trapped air being forced past the plugs by the contraction of chest muscles. The whole process is exhausting and quite frightening, both to observer and victim.

Asthma attacks may be mild and infrequent or they can be exceedingly severe, frequent and sometimes continuous. Severe attacks may require hospitalization. The attack is often proceeded by:

- Coughing, Sneezing, a stuffy or runny nose
- Yawing
- Itching
- The attack itself is characterized by
- Choking and Wheezing
- Straining Chest and Neck Muscles
- Racing Pulse
- Pale Face and Blue Lips
- Face and Body covered with sweat
- A Frightening Sensation of Suffocating.

Foods most often indicted as the villains in asthma vary with age. In infants, milk is probably the number–one cause. In older children and adults, eggs, corn, wheat, chocolate, nuts, peas, beans and peanuts can be causes of asthma reactions.

Allergic Rhinitis

While pollens and sometimes molds are responsible for seasonal rhinitis (hay fever), allergy to food may well be the culprit in perennial allergic rhinitis, with nasal symptoms occurring at any time of year. A victim of this type of allergy symptom has one cold after another, a constant sniffle especially noticeable in the morning and a constant postnasal drip.

Briefly, in perennial rhinitis, the allergen–antibody conflict affects the mucous membrane of the nose, causing swelling (and thus obstruction) and an excessive production of mucus. The following symptoms are common:

- Stuffy nose but blowing is usually unproductive
- Running nose
- Itching of Nose, Eyes and Roof of Mouth
- Excessive Watering of Eyes
- Sneezing and Coughing, also usually unproductive
- Headaches

Besides being a first class nuisance, perennial rhinitis can lead to complications such as sinusitis because the swelling of the nasal membranes can block drainage of the sinuses and prepare the ground for infection. When the sinuses are involved, the victim often suffers from headache, postnasal drip, sometimes fever and sometimes asthma.

Foods most commonly blamed for allergic rhinitis are eggs, milk, wheat, chocolate, beans, peas, tomatoes, onions, salmon, beef, rye, potatoes and citrus fruits–a full market basket of possibilities. Strong odors from such foods as fish, coffee, asparagus milk and from foods cooking may also precipitate allergic rhinitis.

Impairment of taste, smell and hearing may accompany allergic rhinitis. Hearing loss can be a serious and possible permanent result of food allergy. Serous otitis is one of the major causes of deafness in childhood, it occurs most frequently in children between the ages of five and ten. It is caused by swelling and blocking in the eustachian tube, which vents the middle ear into the pharynx. When an allergic reaction causes edema in this tube, fluid accumulates in the middle ear and interferes with hearing. If the allergy is controlled, hearing is usually restored, but permanent damage can occur. Of course hearing loss can be caused by conditions other than food allergy.

Cardiovascular System

Many people do not realize that the heart itself, as well as blood vessels can react allergically, particularly to food allergens. Some allergists believe that cardiac allergic reactions are quite common but usually so mild as to be scarcely noticeable. More severe reactions such as tachycardia (abnormal rapid heart action), anginal pain and even occlusion (closure of a heart blood vessel) have been documented. In some cases, angina pectoris seems to have been controlled by eliminating allergic foods.

Cutaneous System

Eruptions of the skin after eating is commonly understood. we have learned that overindulgence in such deletable things such as chocolate ,cake and ice cream must be paid for by pimples and a marred complexion. We grow wary in our adolescence of such goodies because so much depends upon a radiant and blooming skin.

Food sensitivities are stamped on our hides mainly by three conditions–eczema, urticaria (hives) and angioedema (giant hives). Inhalants, Bacterial agents and Drugs can also be the villains. Physical allergy to heat, cold and light may also bring out such symptoms hives especially.

Allergic Eczema

Allergic eczema due to food can begin at any time of life, but it is more common in infancy and usually can be blamed on cow's milk. Even in old age, eczema can appear, with its scratching and digging. Food seems the number one cause of allergic eczema in infancy. As the child grows older, his problem may become complicated by allergy to inhalants and drugs as well. Or all his symptoms may disappear for awhile only to be replaced by a new allergy, say, to house dust or animal dander or pollen, often with symptoms of allergic rhinitis and asthma. *This rather common progression of allergy in children from colic to eczema to asthma is called the "allergic march." Milk and eggs may be the agents that start it all in the first place, with cereal next in importance.*

Allergic eczema is characterized by diffuse redness with usually a pimply appearance. It commonly shows up on the cheeks, on the ears, in the folds of arms and legs, and on the back and upper part of the body. Once established, it tends to persist indefinitely, subsiding to a tiny patch, then flaring up to cover a good part of the body.

It is thought that allergens are carried to the skin via the blood system and that an inflammatory reaction is set off when allergens and antibodies clash. Itching is the major symptom. Unfortunately, they can predispose the skin to infection, which needless to say, may make matters a great deal worse. Unfortunately, too the itching seems worse at night, so that loss of sleep adds its toll to the victim's suffering. Thus, it is common for the individual with long standing eczema to present a picture of nervousness, irritability, fatigue and sometimes even bizarre behavior.

As with other symptoms of allergy, controversy clouds the role of food in eczema. One school believes that food is the major cause not only in infants but in older children and adults. Another school proclaims that after the first two or three years of life, inhalants are the major source of trouble. As a matter of fact, both factors seem so often to go hand that both usually must be considered and controlled before eczema will exit the scene.

In any case, it seems safe to say that recurrent allergic eczema that peaks from fall to early spring has a good chance of being caused by sensitivity to food, although house dust may be the offender and must be ruled out. If eczema occurs only during the pollen season, it seems reasonable to assume that inhalants are at work. If the itching and lesions follow the administration of a drug (either orally, by injection or topically as a salve or ointment), then eczema clearly results from a drug allergy, Chemicals and other contactants (allergens we touch) can also produce dermatitis (inflammation of the skin) and so have a clear relationship to eczema.

Foods most often indicted in childhood eczema are Milk, Eggs and probably Wheat. In adult eczema these foods, plus oranges, potatoes, spinach and codfish seem to be the most active agents.

Urticaria

Without too much equivocation we can say that sensitivity to food is the most frequent cause of urticaria (hives) in childhood and in adolescence and adulthood, may be as an important agent for this skin reaction as are drugs and chemicals. Inhalants may also cause hives, but probably less commonly that the unholy three of Milk, Eggs and Wheat. Parasitic infestation, toxic conditions and other factors may also produce urticaria as well as angioedema (giant hives) but the largest percentage of these skin manifestations are probably allergic in nature and are normally accompanied by other symptoms of allergy, such as hay fever, asthma, gastrointestinal distress and headaches.

Urticaria can be either acute, with hives appearing at once or almost at once after ingestion of food and lasting for only a short time, or chronic, with hives appearing some time after ingestion and persisting for longer than a month. Uncommon foods such as shellfish, seasonal fruits, nuts and peanuts are apt to be responsible for chronic hives.

In general, the following foods are most often involved in the allergic reactions of both urticaria and angioedema

Fresh Fruits and Vegetables	Nuts
Chocolate	**Peas**
Eggs	**Pork**
Milk	**Wheat**
Wheat	**Fish**
Shellfish	

Those that less commonly bring forth hives are:

- *Beans*
- *Cheese*
- *Corn*
- *Mint and Licorice*
- *Pickles*
- *Mayonnaise and Mustard*
- *Seasonings and Spices*
- *Cola.*

Even the odor of some foods, especially onions and garlic and the cooking fumes of such foods as fish may cause the severely hypersensitive to blossom forth.

More recently indicted by many allergists as agents of urticaria are various additives in food products, particularly dyes of coal tar derivation used to color foods and some preservatives such as benzoic acid and sulfur dioxide

Urticarial Wheals are often haloed in red and look something like mosquito bites with centers. They are characterized by itching and burning. They are commonly widespread over the body and are found especially in areas where clotting exerts pressure.

The mechanism of both urticaria and angioedema are like that of eczema, is still somewhat mysterious, but it is thought that, at least in the acute form, histamine is released to cause blood vessels to dilate and fluid to leak into the tissues. Dilation and leakage are responsible for the redness and swelling. Both types of hives occur frequently in association with visceral symptoms such as abdominal pain and serum sickness like with vomiting, diarrhea, headache and breathing difficulties. Often it takes two allergenic factors working together to produce both these skin reaction.

Angioedema

Angioedema, or Giant Hives, is a strange and sometimes require action to allergens. Regular, recurrent attacks with intervals of relief indicate that food is probably the root of the problem. Edema in this reaction can be quite mild or very severe. When it affects the larynx and mouth, serious obstruction of the airways results. Angioedema can occur in almost any part of the body and in various organs–salivary glands, nerve tissue, membranes of the brain and spinal cord, the gastrointestinal subsystem to list a few. An odd reaction to food is a generalized edema affecting the whole body or at least a good part of it.

Urinary System

It may be helpful to parents to know that food allergy is considered one possible cause of bed wetting and enuresis (the involuntary discharge of urine from the bladder). One study reports that 5 percent of allergic children suffer from enuresis. Cystitis (inflammation of the bladder). Though it can be caused by infection, can also be a reaction to food allergens. And allergy to inhalants can also bring on these problems. But the following foods seem to be the more common agent:

- Eggs
- Milk
- Chocolate
- Food Colors and Flavorings
- Citrus Fruits
- Cola Drinks
- Some Nuts

Sometimes bladder reaction are seasonal, corresponding either with the ingestion of seasonal foods or with pollen or mold spore productions.

Nervous System

Headaches

Allergic headaches are perhaps the most annoying and often the most painful of food allergy manifestations. Just about everyone, children and adults alike are familiar with the torment a headache can cause, but few realize that allergy is often the instigator of their pain. There are, ofcourse other possible causes for headaches–acute and chronic infection (of the sinuses in particular), diseases of the nervous system, brain tumors, heart and liver problems, tension and emotional troubles and others. Normally, headaches with an allergic basis are accompanied by other allergic symptoms such as Rhinitis or Gastrointestinal disturbances Nausea, Vomiting, Diarrhea and Abdominal Distention. But sometimes an aching head is the only symptoms.

The pain or ache of an allergic headache is usually situated along the front of the head, even along the bridge of the nose and cheek area, although it may be felt at the top or back of the head. About 80 percent of frontal headaches are due to allergic causes. Dizziness and sometimes Visual Disorders such as blind areas often accompany an aching head. In fact some pretty bizarre manifestation can occur. How can an allergy to food (or other allergens) cause such distress?

Two things that happen during other types of allergic reaction can also happen in the cranial area:

1. Edema due to the leakage of fluid from blood vessels dilating and thinning in response to the allergen antibody conflict, and
2. Constriction or Spasm of the smooth muscles.

The Nausea and Vomiting that can accompany allergic headaches is probably the allergy process. It is generally believed that emotions and stress play a part in allergic headaches, probably as a trigger rather than as a primary agent. And, of course an allergic headache itself can produce emotional symptoms of disorientation and confusion.

Opinion is divided as the relative importance of food and inhalants in allergic headache. One food or several may be the agents of these headaches and an additional allergy to an inhalant can complicate matters. The onset of pain may not immediately follow the ingestion of an allergenic food but may arrive hours later. The following foods are most commonly responsible for allergic headaches:

- Nuts
- Chocolate
- Milk
- Wheat
- Corn
- Fish
- Citrus fruit
- Eggs
- Tomatoes

Sinus Headache

Sinus Headache is a term loosely applied to headaches characterized by frontal pain and pain around the eyes. Sinus headaches can be caused by allergic rhinitis and its concomitant edema and congestion. Unless accompanied by a thick, yellowish nasal discharge and local tenderness, the chances are that such a headache is not the infectious condition of true sinusitis.

Migraine

Migraine meaning half head seems to be a disease that plagues only the "civilized". Perhaps the most mysterious of all headaches is migraine

Migraine headaches may begin in childhood; but most often they appear in early adulthood. Somewhere around half the victims reported that it runs in their families. Certainly, most of us have known at least one person who retires periodically to a darkened room to wait out the storm of this extremely painful affliction.

Some doctors believe that sensitivity to food is a major cause; others discount the role of allergy altogether. Still others believe that the percentage of migraine due to allergy is about the same as the percentage of allergic persons in the total population.

Migraine typically makes its presence felt about one to three times a month. In between attacks the victim is entirely free of symptoms. Sometimes attacks are preceded by an aura, a disturbance of the senses ranging from vague feelings of tension to visual distortions such as flashing bright lights. The victims may even hear noises. Usually migraine arrives in the morning and rapidly mushrooms into a pounding ache, perhaps generalized at first but then localized in one area of the head. It may or may not be accompanied by nausea, vomiting and other symptoms of gastrointestinal distress. Normally all this misery lasts from about eight to twenty four hours, but it can linger for several days.

Migraine can be triggered by physical agents such as cold, heat and light, or by tension, stress and fatigue, or by gastrointestinal upsets and infections. The following foods are thought to play a major role.

Eggs milk
Wheat pork
Fish chocolate
Legumescorn
Garlic cinnamon

In addition, individuals suffering this unhappy condition would do well to avoid alcoholic beverages, particularly red wine and champagne. They may also have to forego aged cheese, especially cheddarcheese, since these contain tyramine, a substance that seems to precipitate migraine.

Histaminic Headache

There is one other type of headache we should mention here the histaminic headache. The relationship of allergy to this rather strange headache is not yet clear. Some doctors believe food allergy is a basic cause, others doubt that allergy has much if anything to do with it. In any case, the headache itself is a "Bummer". It is of very brief duration. Lasting usually only for a few minutes. But those few minutes can be terrifying. The headache often arrives at night, bringing a sound sleeper bolt upright as if he had been stabbed. The pain is so intense that usually he is forced to walk around until it subsides. It is a piercing, burning pain, often on one side of the head at one time, on the other side at another time. It can also occur in the general area of the frontal or eye and sometimes in the face. The headache seems to result from the release of histamine with dilation of intracranial and extracranial blood vessels. Fortunately, histaminic headache is uncommon.

Allergic Tension- Fatigue Syndrome

The mechanism of allergic tension fatigue syndrome like that of migraine is open to speculation. Some allergists believe that it is a definite allergic reaction of localizededemain nerve and other tissue, occurring by itself or accompanied by other allergic symptoms, such as eczema, hay fever and asthma.

The symptoms of the allergic tension, fatigue syndromeare the following.

- Drowsiness and Inability to concentrate
- Fatigue and Listlessness
- Confusion
- Depression
- Emotional Instability and Irritability
- Belligerence
- Poor Coordination
- Temper Tantrums and Schizophrenic Manifestation (Occasionally)

Foods Most Often Indicted are

- Milk
- Wheat
- Spices and condiments
- Eggs
- Chocolate
- Cola

Epilepsy

It is now believed by some allergists that a certain percentage of epilepsy cases may be due to allergy, in all probability to food allergy. Some doctors even believe that allergy may be the major cause of this strange disorder others insist the percentage in very small.

Emotional Disturbance

While allergy to food may be responsible for a good many of the specific symptoms of the nervous system. Other symptoms of sensitivity to food may be so severe as to trail emotional and psychological problems in their wake. Thus, allergy to food (or whatever)can be either directly an agent of emotional disturbances or indirectly, because of the anguish it causes.

CHAPTER VII

SYMPTOMS OF FOOD ALLERGY

There are no immunological methods for accurately confirming or predicting the allergic symptoms that may follow ingestion of any food. The reactions may occur in almost any body system–gastrointestinal, respiratory, cutaneous, urinary, or nervous system, mucous glands, and mucous membranes.

Common Allergic Symptoms

System	Symptoms
Gastro intestinal	Canker Sores, Cheilitis, Colic, Colitis, Diarrhea, Malabsorption, Enteropathy, Vomiting.
Respiratory	Rhinitis, Cough, Asthma, Bronchitis
Cutaneous	Angioedema, Eczema, Pruritus, Purpura, Urticaria.
Central Nervous System	Headache, Neuralgias, Irritability Personality change.
Miscellaneous	Pallor, Enuresis, Retarded Growth Menstrual Irregularity

Manifestations of allergy may occur in any part of the body. The tissues of these systems are frequently involved. Cutaneous, Gastrointestinal, Respiratory and Neurological. The symptoms are consequently varied depending on the parts affected.

1. Skin Manifestations may include Cancer Sores, Dermatitis, Edema, Fever Blisters, Pruritus and Urticarial (Hives).

2. Common Gastrointestinal manifestations include Cheilitis, Stomatitis, Colic in Infants, Abdominal Distention, Constipation, Diarrhea, Dyspepsia, and Nausea and Vomiting. The symptoms may be suggestive of Appendicitis, Colitis, Gallbladder Disease or Ulcers, and there may be confusion in diagnosis.

3. Respiratory symptoms include Allergic Rhinitis, Asthma, Bronchitis and Nasal Polyps among others.

4. Neurologic symptoms such as Migraine, Neuralgias and the Tension–Fatigue Syndrome are sometimes due to food allergy. The latter syndrome characterized by Anxiety, Fatigue, Irritability, Muscle and Joint Aching, Restlessness, Stomach Pains and so on.

5. Miscellaneous symptoms such as Anaphylactic Reactions, Arthralgias, Arthritis, and Edema have been attributed to Food Allergy

Gastrointestinal

- Abdominal Pain
- Nausea
- Vomiting

- Diarrhea
- Gastro intestinal Bleeding
- Protein–Losing Enteropathy
- Oral and Pharyngeal Pruritus

Cutaneous

- Urticaria
- Eczema
- Angioedema
- Erythema
- Itching

Respiratory

- Rhinitis
- Asthma
- Cough
- Milk – induced syndrome with respiratory disease (Heiner's syndrome)

Systemic

- Anaphylaxis
- Hypotension

Controversial or Unproven

- Behavioral Conditions
- Tension-Fatigue Syndrome
- Attention Deficit Hyperactivity Disorder
- Otitis media.
- Psychiatric Disorders
- Neurologic Disorders
- Neurologic Disorders
- Musculoskeletal Disorders
- Migraine Headache

The Spectrum of Food Allergic Reactions

1. *Cow's Milk Allergy*

They found that the patients could be divided into-three groups. First, those children who showed immediate symptoms with small amounts of milk, evidenced by anaphylaxis, angio-oedema, urticaria and diarrhoea; secondly, those who developed symptoms often up to several hours after intake of moderate amounts of milk (approximately 200ml) and in whom the skin test to the offending food was generally negative; and thirdly, those mostly older children suffering from a poorly defined multisystem involvement, including e.g.skin, lung ,gastro intestinal tract, central nervous system (migraine), who often required larger amounts more frequently and in whom symptoms could take well over 24 hours to occur)

2. *Atopic Eczema*

Eczema can occur in exclusively breastfed infants and this can be due to the transfer of absorbed food antigens from the mother's diet to her milk. Food intolerance and enhanced immune responsiveness to foods are also features of atopic eczema in adults. The antigens concerned are usually in fish, shellfish, eggs, peanuts, tree nuts and milk. Sensitivity to the latter does not seem to be frequent in childhood. A possible role of the skin and other immunological sites during primary food antigen sensitization is likely.

3. *Asthma*

Asthma overall is an important risk factor in patients suffering food allergic and in particular anaphylactic reactions. In about 5% of patients with asthma, foods may cause worsening of their symptoms.

4. *Cow's Milk – Sensitive Colitis*

Typically an infant with food sensitive colitis presents before the age of 1 year, with loose stools containing mucus and blood. An elimination diet and clinical monitoring with Rectal Biopsy shows a pattern of improvement similar to that seen clinically. The pathology of the rectum differs from classic ulcerative colitis in that there is preservation of the architecture of the mucosal crypts, with no crypt abscess formation and no depletion of goblet cell mucus.

Chapter VIII

Clinical Manifestations of Food Allergy

Mechanisms of Allergy and Food Intolerance

The immunological principle of an allergic response will be reviewed briefly.

The offending substance, called the allergen or antigen, may gain access to the body by, ingestion, inhalation, direct contact of injection (drugs, serum). The allergen, usually a protein passes through the gastrointestinal mucosa (in the case of a food allergy) and is perceived by the host's immune system in the body's circulation. The first time the antigen appears in the circulation there is no clinical allergic response to it, but it stimulates the production of antibodies(Ab) one or more classes of immunoglobulins (Ig): IgA, IgE., IgG or IgM. The antibodies remain attached to cells or circulate in the body. The nest time the antigen (Ag) appears in the circulation, it will form a complex with its specific antibody, and these complexes may then act on serum and cells to give the biological effects of an allergic reaction. Allergic responses include the production of anaphylatoxins, kines or histamine, which can cause inflammatory reaction and shock. Individual organs respond in different ways to the antigen–antibody complexes.

IgA, which coats the intestinal tract, seems to be somewhat protective against the development of food allergy. Practically speaking, if highly allergenic foods are into introduced until after an infant has developed intestinal IgA (age 7 months), food allergies are less likely to develop. Before this age the infant's gastrointestinal tract is more permeable to dietary proteins, which may enter circulation and stimulate the production of antibodies.

In addition to this antibody component of the immune reaction, the body also contains a cellular component that does not depend on antibodies. This type of reaction is sometimes referred to as delayed hyper sensitivity.

The role of cellular immunity in food allergy reaction is still unclear, but it may account for a chronic allergic response and stress state the allergic tension–fatigue syndrome. The person, usually a child, has the typical allergic look, dull faces, infraorbital circles and an allergic gape. Symptoms that occur immediately after ingestion of a certain food obviously are easier to diagnose as being due to food allergy than are delayed symptoms such as diarrhoea. Uncooked foods are more likely to induce immediate allergic reactions. A delayed reaction may be caused by one of the digestive products of the food, which would explain why the patient may not have positive response to skin test using the whole food.

Manifestations

Several manifestation of allergy may appear in the same individual, varying from a minor reaction such as slight eye or nose itching or rash to severe gastrointestinal symptoms such as diarrhea, vomiting and cramping. Stunted growth and malnutrition are sometimes traced to an allergy. Bronchial asthma, hay fever, dermatitis, urticaria, eczema, acne, migraine headaches, canker sores and cardiovascular disorders are some of the observed manifestation of an allergy that may be caused by foods, anorexia and food aversion may be the to an allergy to one or more common foods Clinical symptoms of food allergy are listed.

They are:

- Colic
- Sniffles that persist
- Abdominal pain
- Diarrhea and/or constipation
- Excessive vomiting
- Skin rashes and eczema
- Cancer sores
- Needs for formula changes and refusal of food in infants fretfulness
- Failure to thrive

Clinical Features of Adverse Reactions Attributed to Food and Food Ingredients

System affected	Clinical features that could be caused by adverse reactions to foods.
Skin	Urticaria Atopic dermatitis Angioedema
Gastrointestinal tract	Oral allergy syndrome (burning, itching of the lips and mouth and sometimes the larynx and pharynx) Pain, colic Nausea Vomiting Change in stool habit e.g. looseness, frequency, blood, mucus Abdominal distension, flatulence Heartburn (gastro-esophageal reflux)
Respiratory tract	Asthma
	Rhinitis
Eyes	Watering eyes Conjunctivitis Periocular pruritus
Cardiovascular system	Symptoms and signs of hypo – and hypertension
Blood	Symptoms and signs of hemolytic anaemia (rare)
Central nervous system	Headache abnormal behavior in children (including attention deficit hyperactivity disorder (ADHD). Fatigue Lassitude
Generalized systemic	Anaphylaxis (circulatory collapse, wheeze, inability swallow and other symptoms)

CHAPTER IX

DIAGNOSIS OF FOOD ALLERGY

No simple Test can be used to diagnose Food Allergy. Diagnosis requires identification of the suspected food, proof that the food causes an adverse response and verification of the immunological involvement, Nonallergic mechanisms must be ruled out. The omission of foods from the diet on the basis of improper diagnosis can threaten nutritional status.

A history is the first tool used in diagnosis. Information gathered includes a description of symptoms, time from ingestion of food to onset of symptoms, a description of the most recent reactions, a list of suspected foods and an estimate of the quantity of food required to produce a reaction. Because food allergy may be linked to the introduction of new foods, early feeding history should be explored. Family history of allergy should also be reviewed.

Physical examination includes measurement of weight and height (and head circumference for the infant). Measurements are plotted on a growth chart and are evaluated in relationship to earlier measurements. Decreased weight for height may be related to malabsorption and food allergy. Therefore, patterns of growth and their relationship to the onset of symptoms should be explored. Clinical signs of malnutrition should be assessed, including the evaluation of fat ad musclestores. Evidence of chronic conditions such as eczema, rhinitis, and asthma are also evaluated.

A food and symptom diary is kept for 1 to 2 weeks and information recorded includes the type of food, the time and amount eaten, the time of appearance of symptoms and the medications taken. Medications may alter the symptoms observed. The food and symptom diary helps to document symptoms and may suggest a relationship to diet that is not apparent from recall. This record also serves as a baseline for future intervention.

Biochemical testing serves to rule out non allergenic causes for symptoms. A complete blood count and differential blood count; tests of stool for reducing substances, ova, and parasite or occult blood and sweat chloride test for the exclusion of cystic fibrosis are examples of tests that may be useful.

Immunologic testing cannot be used to diagnose food allergy but can help to identify suspected foods and to confirm an immunological mechanism. Positive immunological test results must be confirmed by an adverse reaction when the food is eaten (Bock et al, 1977). Reliable reactions should continue to be monitored during this time.

Food challenges may precipitate anaphylactic reactions (David, 1984). To minimize risks to patients, all challenges that may cause an anaphylactic reaction should be carried out in a physician's office or hospital. The initial dose is increased in a stepwise fashion over 1 hour until a reaction is observed or a total of 8 to 10 grams of dried food has been consumed. The patient is then observed for an additional 2 hours before discharge. If there is clear history of a life threatening anaphylactic reaction after eating a specific food, it should not be challenged (Sampson, 1988). A double–bind food challenge can be used when symptoms are subjective, when multiple food allergies have been suggested, or when psychosocial components are suspected. For the older child and adult who are able to swallow capsules, dried food is placed in opaque capsules. For the child who is not able to swallow capsules, the suspected food is concealed in a food or beverage known to be tolerated, such as apple Sause, juice, or a specially prepared cookie. Capsules or masking foods are administered twice per challenge. On one occasion the individual receives the food being tested. On the other, a placebo is given. In a double- blind food challenge neither the person administering the challenge nor the person being challenged knows which has been offered. A single–blind food challenge, in which the person receiving the challenge does not know what has been offered, may be useful in similar situations and is easier to implement. Challenges carried out for research purpose, should be double–blind (Bock, 1986; Sampson, 1988).

Diagnostic Tests

Type of Test	Description	Comments
Skin testing(scratch, prick, or puncture)	A drop of antigen is placed skin, which is the scratched punctured To allow penetration	Most sensitive test but over diagnoses food allergy; should be followed by food challenge
Radioallergosorbent test (RAST)	Serum mixed with food on paper disk and then washed with radioactively labeled IgE	No more accurate than skin test but more costly; may be useful for people who have had anaphylaxis or who have skin disease.
CAP-RAST fluorescein-enzyme immunoassay(FEIA)	Compared to RAST, this test binds more allergen	New test for food allergy,availed for only six foods as of October 1988; shows promise as a component in diagnostic process for food allergy
Enzyme LinkedImmunosorbent Assay(ELISA)	Much like RAST, except no radioactive material used	Same as RAST
Cytotoxic testing	Allergen mixed with whole blood or serum leukocyte suspension; lysed leukocytes are counted	Unreliable
Sublingual testing	Drops of allergen extract placed under the Tongue and symptoms are recorded	Unreliable
Provocation testing and neutralization	Subcutaneous injection of extract elicits symptoms followed by weaker or stronger injection to neutralize symptoms	Unreliable
Kinesiologic testing	Arm extended and foods to be tested placed in hand; test is positive if arm moves more easily after food has been placed in hand.	Unreliable

Diagnosis of Food Allergy

1. History
2. Frequency, Type, Severity, Seasonality of Reactions, Interval since Food Ingestion, Coexisting Intestinal Disease.
3. Clinical Examination
4. Entity, Degree, Extension, Overlap of symptoms
   - In Vivo Tests
5. Skin Prick Test
6. Elimination Diet
7. Open Challenge
8. Double Blind Placebo Controlled Challenge
9. Gastrointestinal Procedures
   - Intestinal permeability evaluation with and without challenge
   - Endoscopy before and after challenge
   - Biopsy
10. In Vitro Tests
11. Food Specific Ig E Antibodies
12. Food Specific IgG Antibodies(only suitable in some cases of monitoring of diabetic compliance).
13. Cellular Tests (Lymphocyte Proliferation)
14. Mediators in Biological Fluids after Food Challenge
15. Histological Examination of Intestinal Biopsy

CHAPTER X

TREATMENT

Allergy-Schematic Diagram

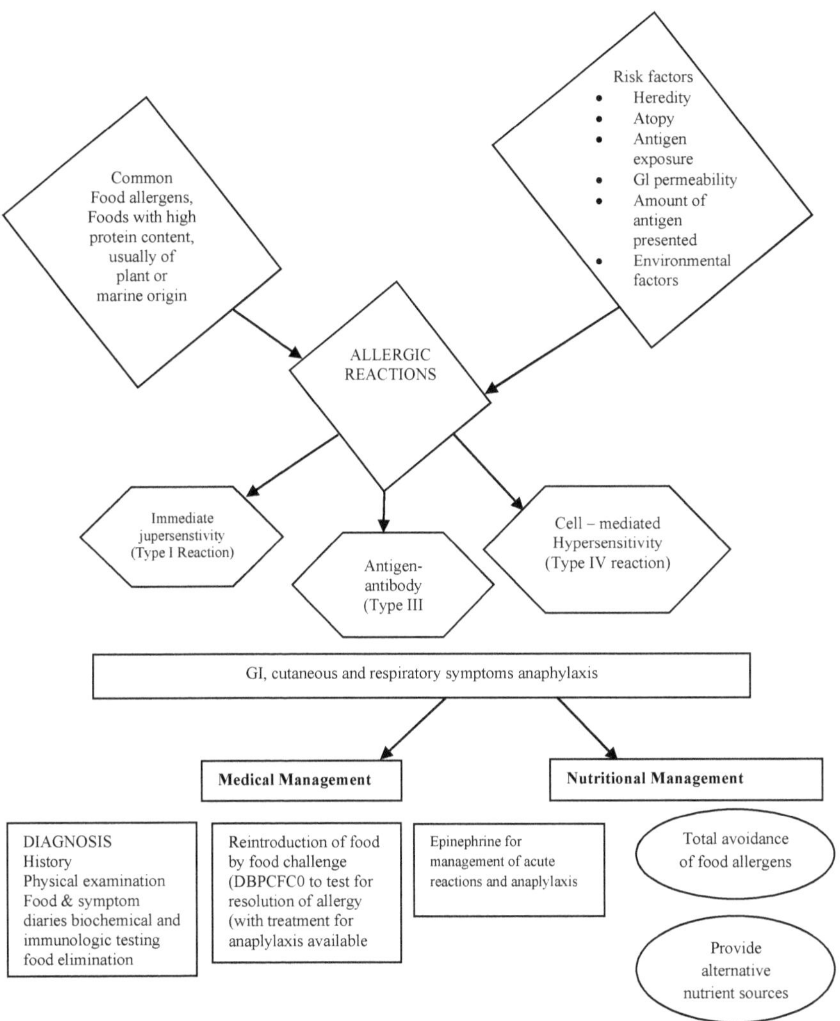

Once the source of the allergy is determined, treatment is that of strict avoidance. The second, and also important, aspect of management involves a careful assessment of the nutritional adequacy of the diet. Comparable foods must be substituted for the foods eliminated, particularly when they represent important sources of energy, protein, vitamins, and minerals. The three allergens which require the most aggressive management in relation and maintaining consistent avoidance are milk, wheat, and egg

1. *Elimination Diets*

Elimination of the Causative Food

If a positive food factor is identified and can be eliminated from the diet, then the symptoms will not recur. For example, if the responsible article of food is one which is not consumed regularly (e.g. shellfish), it can easily be avoided. It is far more difficult in the case of eggs, milk and wheat which are present in so many foods–cakes, puddings, sauces, gravies soups, etc. Give a full list of articles of diet to be avoided if a patient is allergic to milk, eggs or wheat. In addition other methods must be tried in such a situations.

Elimination diets have a proper place in the diagnosis and management of food intolerance. In elimination diets, the suspected food is excluded in the daily diet.

The common elimination diets are:

(i) **Simple exclusion diets**: When a single food like milk, egg or wheat is suspected, patients are advised how to consume a diet free of these. This is not simple in practice. Exclusion of foods like milk in children, require expertise to ensure that dietary requirements are met.

(ii) **Multi Exclusion diet**: if it is not clear from dietary enquiry or simple exclusion diet which foods are responsible, a complex exclusion and has to be tried on trial and error basis.

    (a) **Initial exclusion diets**: Initially a wide range of foods which may provoke intolerance is removed from diet and after a period of time, reintroduced singly into the diet so the offending item is identified.

    (b) **Graduated exclusion diet**: The number of foods excluded from a diet is gradually increased. One should read the labels carefully for 'under cover' allergens. While cooling, one should avoid any cross – contact between the food allergen and foods prepared without the allergenic ingredient. It is better to avoid all processed foods which contain many.

Two Stages of Elimination Diets

Elimination Diet -1 Milk, Egg and Wheat Free

Food sources	Allowed	Avoid
Animal protein sources vegetable protein sources Grains or alternate	Lamb, chicken, turkey, beef, pork soy milk, soy beans, other beans, lentils, peanuts white potato, sweet potato, yams, rice, tapioca, arrowroot, buckwheat, corn, barley, rye, millet, oats	Cow's milk chicken eggs Wheat
Vegetables	All vegetables	
Fruits	All fruits and juices	
Sweeteners	Cane or beet sugar, maple syrup, corn syrup	
Oils	Soy oil, corn oil, safflower oil, coconut oil, vegetable oil, olive oil, peanut oil, milk-free margarines	Butter and margarines that include milk.
Other	Salt, all spices	

Elimination Diet -2 Milk, Egg and Wheat- Free

Sources	Allowed	Avoid
Animal protein sources	Lamb	All other animal protein : meat, fish, poultry, eggs, and milk
Vegetable protein sources		Soymilk, soy beans, peas, other beans, lentils, peanuts, bean sprouts, all nuts
Grains or alternate Starches	White potato, sweet potato, yams, rice, tapioca, buckwheat, arrowroot	Wheat, oats, corn, barely, millet, rye
Vegetables	All vegetables except corn, peas, tomatoes	Com, peas, tomatoes
Fruits	All fruits and juices except citrus fruits strawberries	Citrus fruits, strawberries
Sweeteners	Cane or beet sugar, maple syrup	Com syrup, com syrup solids
Oils	Safflower oil, coconut oil, olive oil, sesame oil	Butter, margarine, vegetable oils, soy oil, corn oil, peanut oil, nonspecific shortening, or fats of animal origin
Others	Salt, pepper, all spices, vanilla or lemon extract, baking soda, cream tartar	Chocolate coffee, tea, colas and other soft drinks, alcoholic beverages corn starch, baking powder with corn starch.

2. *Denaturation of Protein*

Denaturation can help allergic activity of food, e.g., patient may be sensitive to raw milk but boiled may be suitable.Sometimes if a protein is denatured by heat it ceases to act as an allergen. Thus a patient sensitive to raw milk or lightly boiled eggs may be able to take with impunity boiled eggs may be able to take with impunity boiled milk or an egg which has been boiled for at least 10 minutes. Patients who are sensitive to eggs may be able to take the yolks, especially if well cooked, although the whites may continue to cause symptoms.

3. *Desensitization*

Many attempts have been made to desensitize patients who suffer from food allergy by repeatedly injecting small quantities of the allergen or giving small amounts by mouth. This method is generally regarded as being of little or no value.

4. *Hypersensitization*

Some physicians have been trying to help patients by giving repeatedly small doses of the allergen either by mouth or injection in the hope that their sensitivity may disappear.

5. *Drugs*

A number of drugs that mitigate the symptoms of allergy are available. Antihistamines are effective in controlling local forms of allergy like urticaria and angioedema. Although drugs causing somnolence are effective, these are likely to cause discomfort when taken regularly. Bronchodilator drugs are effective in treatment of bronchial spasms in attacks of asthma. Corticosteroids are highly effective in prevention of attacks. Compared with the complexity of diagnosis, the prevention is straightforward. Neither immunotherapy nor oral desensitization has proved successful in preventing allergic reaction to food. Although many foods are easily avoided, some may be taken inadvertently in concealed form; complications of avoidance may include growth retardation, vitamin deficiency disorders and impairment of musculature. These sequelae of long term nutritional deprivation are preventable.

Adrenaline and its derivatives are useful in allergic asthma and anaphylactic shock, and corticosteroids for the alleviation of the immediate symptoms of allergic shock. However the danger of long term corticosteroid therapy severely limits their use. The prescription of tranquillizers and sedatives is often indicated because of the close connection between emotion and allergy, but no drug is capable of bringing about desensitization.

Allergies can also be caused by inhaling pollen, cosmetic of perfumes.

Allergic reactions can adversely affect a child's nutritional status and health. The solution may not be easy but can be found by identifying the allergen.

6. *Milk Free Diet*

Since milk is the primary source of nutrients in infancy and continues to function as a valuable contributor of protein energy, calcium, and riboflavin during childhood and into adult life, the child with milk allergy requires special consideration. The milk–sensitive infant may be given one of the soybean or hypoallergenic milk substitutes. Some children who are sensitive to the lactalbumin in milk may be able to tolerate goat's, milk as a substitute because the whey portion, which is the lactalbumin portion is different in goat's milk and cow's milk. It is important to note, however, that a macrocytic anemia due to a deficiency of vitamin B in goat's milk sometimes occurs in the children receiving this substitute.

Type of food	Foods allowed	Foods avoided
Beverages	Carbonated drinks, fruit juices, cocoa made with water, lemonade, tea, special formulas	Fresh, dried, or evaporated milk, malted milk, cocoa made with milk solids.
Bread and crackers	French bread, rye bread, homemade bread made without milk, pretzels, Ritz crackers, Biscuit, graham crackers, saltines, soda premium.	Bread unless made without milk; hot breads (pancakes, waffles, griddle cakes, muffins, biscuits)
Cereals	Any cereal served with fruit juice or milk substitute	Cereals if served with milk or cream.
Meals, fish, and poultry	All, if prepared without sauces made with milk or cream.	Wieners and bologna if milk solids added in processing (check labels)
Eggs	In any form, if milk is not added	None, if milk is not added
Cheese	None	In all forms
Desserts	Fruit, fruited Jell-O, homemade puddings made without milk (tapioca, junket, cornstarch pudding), fruit ice, water ice, homemade pies, cakes, cookies made without milk.	Ice cream, sherbet, all pudding, custards cakes, pies, and cookies made with milk, yogurt
Fats	Vegetable oils, lard, margarines without added milk solids (kosher margarine)	Butter, cream, sour cream margarine with added milk solids salad dressings with milk added
Potato and substitutes	Potato, rice, pastas (spaghetti, macaroni, noodles) if milk or cheese is not added	None, if milk, cream, butter, or cheese is not added.
Soups	Broth, clear consumer, bouillon broth – based	Creamed soups
Vegetables	All	None, if milk, cream, butter, or cheese is not added
Fruits	All	None
Miscellaneous	Moderate amounts of sugar, jams, jellies, lollipops, bard candies, peanut butter, nuts, corn chips potato chips, popcorn (without butter added). Pickles olives, meat juice gravy	Candy made with milk (caramels, milk chocolate, fondant, nougat), hollandaise sauce.

7. *Wheat Free Diet*

Since most baked and commercial products use wheat flour as an important ingredient, strict adherence to a wheat–free diet is a particular challenge. Obtaining an adequate energy intake is often difficult on this regimen. The avoidance of enriched wheat flour removes a good source of iron, thiamin, niacin, and riboflavin from the child, and care must be taken to ensure that these nutrients are provided from other sources. Rice flour may be substituted in most recipes, in the proportion of ¾ cup of rice flour for 1 cup of regular wheat flour.

Type of food	Foods allowed	Foods avoided
Beverages	Milk, carbonated drinks, fruit juices lemonade, hot chocolate	Postum, Ovaltine
Breadand crackers	Rye bread if 100% rye, Crisp corn bread or muffins, rice flour bread or muffins if made at home without wheat flour added	All other breads, rolls, crackers
Cereals	Any corn, oat, or rice cereal	Wheat cereals –farina, bran, puffed wheat, shredded wheat
Meat, fish and poultry	Plain meats, fish, and poultry prepared without breading and without gravy made with flour	Breaded meats, processed meats (wieners, hot dogs) if bread fillers added, meat loaf, croquettes meatballs if bread added
Eggs	Fired, poached, boiled scrambled, baked	None
Cheese	Cheddar, American, Swiss, cottage, farmer	None, unless flour is added to processed cheese foods.
Desserts	Fruits, Jell-O, fruit ice, sherbet, ice cream, custard, junket, pudding made from rice or cornstarch	Cakes, pies, flour is added to processed cheese foods.
Fats	Vegetable oils, butter, margarine, lard	Salad dressings, gravy, if thickened with flour
Potatoand substitutes	Potato, rice	Spaghetti, noodles, macaroni, stuffing unless made with rice, dumplings
Soups	Homemade soups, consommé, made without	All canned soups
Vegetables	All	Only if sauce made with flour is added
Fruits	All	None
Miscellaneous	Moderate amounts of sugar, jams, jellies, peanut butter, nuts potato, chips pickles, olives, meat juice gravy	Beer, pretzels.

8. *Egg Free Diet*

Egg has many uses in cooking and therefore its presence in foods is extremely common. Other foods rich in protein and iron such as meat, fish, and poultry, can be substituted for egg. The primary nutritional concern in the growing child who is egg-sensitive therefore relates to ensuring adequate calories, since a great majority of baked goods contain egg and need to be avoided. Egg is used as a binder and to add volume to cakes, as a thickening agent in creamed dishes and sauces, to help pies and cookies brown, and as a glaze for breads. To replace a egg as the binding substance in cakes, an equal amount of mashed banana may be substituted. An extra ½ teaspoon of baking powder can also be added to the egg-free cake recipe to make up for the loss of volume.

Types of food	Foods allowed	Foods avoided
Beverages	All except those which have egg added.	Eggnog
Breadand crackers	Saltine crackers, soda crackers, graham crackers, white, wheat, rye French. Pumper nicked breads.	Hot breads or any breads and crackers made with egg, French toast.
Cereals	Any	None
Meat, fish, and poultry	All except those with egg added	Any prepared or coated with egg; sausage, croquettes, meat loaf
Eggs	None	All
Cheese	All	None
Desserts	Fruits, Jelly, Fruit ice, sherbet, ice cream, puddings if made without egg, pies if made without egg.	Cakes, cookies, frostings, French ice cream made with eggs, meringue, custards, Bavarian creams
Fats	Vegetable oils, butter, margarine, lard	Salad dressing if egg added
Potatoand substitutes	Potato, rice noodles except those with added egg, macaroni, spaghetti	Egg noodles
Soups	All except those with egg or egg noodles added	Soups with egg or egg noodles
Vegetables	All	None
Fruits	All	None
Miscellaneous	Moderate amounts of sugar, jams, jellies, peanut butter, nuts potato, chips pickles, olives, meat juice gravy	Hollandaise sauce, candies made with egg.

9. *Substitution of Alternative Foods*

This is sometimes possible in the case of milk. A child sensitive to cow's milk may not necessarily be sensitive to goat's milk. There are proprietary preparations of soya bean which can be used as a substitute for milk. Similarly a child sensitive to wheat may do well on oats, rice or barley.

10. Diet Counselling

Patients who are sensitive to eggs may be able to take egg yolk as egg white is the main allergen. Patient allergic to particular food should avoid it for at least a period of time. After six months, it can be tried but with great caution, if it is an important article in diet. The patient should be able to recognize the offending food and should inform the doctor before treatment and diagnosis.

Food allergies are often inherited and almost all are identified early in life. Infants are much more likely to have food allergies than adults and many allergies are outgrown. Milk allergy is usually outgrowth by age three. The changed reactivity can be due to the decreased absorption of immunologic food proteins as the intestinal mucosa and the secretory immune system mature. Based primarily upon studies performed in the United States in children older than two years of age, egg, milk, peanut, tree nuts and fish are the common allergies

Successful treatment depends on good counseling based on the following considerations.

A thorough diet history must serve as the basis for counseling.

1. When an important nutrient source or an entire food group must be eliminated because of the allergy, alternate food sources must be included.
2. Special help with food selection must be given. Prepared, processed, and mixed dishes often are a particular hazard. Shopping for foods must be done with a careful eye on labels. Also, guidelines for restaurant choices and other meals eaten away from home are important for proper treatment.
3. Another area of concern is advice regarding recipes appropriate for milk-free, wheat free, and egg-free diets.
4. A thorough diet history must serve as the basis for counseling.
5. In certain instances it may be necessary to supplement the diet with vitamin or mineral preparations (e.g., calcium) or both, if alternative food sources cannot be successful added.
6. Strict avoidance of the food allergen and relied of the troubles symptoms are vital concerns in the management of food allergy, but also necessary is a sensitivity to the nutritional and emotional needs of the child. Nutritional adequacy, interest, and variety are important goals in the food allergy diet included.

11. *Maintaining the Nutrition of the Patient*

Many intelligent allergic patients, knowing something of the nature of their disease, go to great lengths to avoid any food that may aggravate it. Some avoid so many kinds of food that they become severely undernourished. A similar result may result may follow from unwise advice from their doctors. This is particularly true in the case of growing children. It must be stressed that allergic patients should not be subjected to dietary restrictions without good evidence that their symptoms are due to a food allergen. In many cases this can only be determined in a clinic where the appropriate tests can be carried out.

12. *Dietary Treatment of Food Allergy*

Especially for children, it is always necessary to consider the relative importance of the allergic disturbance in relation to the diet. It is better management, for example, to treat a mild case of eczema locally than to subject the child to the dangers of an inadequate diet with its far more serious consequences.

If a single food such as strawberries or grapefruit is implicated, the food is easily omitted from the diet. If allergy involves more than one food, the initial diet contains only those foods that produce no reactions. Thus, if improvement has occurred on an elimination diet, simple, not mixed, foods are added, one at a time, to the allowed list of foods. Several days to a week must elapse between the additions of each new food. A given food should be tested on at least two, preferably three, occasions before it is permanently added to, or eliminated from, the diet. Because wheat, eggs, and milk are frequent allergens, these foods are added last.

Dietary adequacy becomes a matter of great concern when important foods are eliminated for a long period of time. This is especially true in infants and young children and care must be taken to ensure inclusion of acceptable foods similar in nutrient content to the one omitted.

In milk sensitivity changing the form of the milk sometimes improvers tolerance that is, boiled, powdered, acidulated, or evaporated milk may be satisfactory when fresh cow's milk is not. Some children will tolerate no milk whatsoever, and a hypoallergenic formula must be substituted. Many youngsters outgrow their sensitivity to milk but others need to continue a milk–free diet indefinitely.

13. Hyposensitization

It consists of decreasing the sensitivity to a given substance by giving minute doses of the allergen in gradually increasing amounts. It is a very tedious procedure and is seldom used in food allergy, and then only when a major food group is involved.

14. Dietary Management for Asthmatic Patients

Those who have severe asthma often find it difficult to consume an adequate diet. The meals should be small and eaten slowly in an environment free from stress. Interval feedings are necessary to bolster the calorie intake. Fluid intake should be encouraged usually breakfast and lunch is the best meals of the day, and particular attention should be paid to their nutritional quality and attractiveness. A rest period after meals is helpful. Ordinarily, late-evening feedings are not advisable. Some clinicians routinely eliminate highly allergenic foods such as chocolate, nuts, shellfish, and so on. Milk products are sometimes omitted because of their tendency to form mucus.

15. Instructing the Patient

Patients who follow an elimination diet program for a long period require careful supervision. It is not sufficient to instruct the patient to omit specific offending foods. The essential, nutritious foods should be included in the diet if possible. If foods such as milk, meat or eggs are eliminated, adequate substitutions or supplements must be made. Malnutrition must be guarded against when the diet is severely restricted.

A number of procedures have been advocated for the treatment of foods to render them less antigenic. One of these procedures is the denaturation of food. This is done by chemical treatment or by heat and is both simple and useful. For example, denatured milk (boiled, evaporated and powdered) is valuable prophylactically

16. Diet in Genetic Disorders

Genes control not only common hereditary characteristics but also the metabolic functions of the cell. When a specific gene is abnormal (mutant) the enzyme whose synthesis it controls cannot be made. In turn, the metabolic reaction controlled by the enzyme cannot take place. A genetic disease would manifest symptoms relative to those reaction products. Phenylketonuria Table gives details of genetic disorders having nutritional implications.

Genetic Disorders having Nutritional Implications

Name of the disorder	Enzyme affected	Nutrient involved and therapy
Phenylketonuria	Phenylalanine hydroxylase	Low protein (phenylalanine) adequate energy.
Maples syrup urine disease	Branded chain ketoacid dehydrogenase complex	Low protein (leucine, isoleucine, valine) adequate energy, and supplemental calcium.
Homocystinural	Cystathoninebetasynthase	Low protein (methionine) and adequate energy and calcium.
Citrullinemia	Arginiosuccinic acid	Low protein, adequate energy, supplemental calcium, vitamin and mineral.
Tryrosinemia	Fumarylaceto-acetate hydrolase	Low protein *tyrosine and phenylalanine) adequate energy.
Galactosaemia	Variant forms, 3 different enzymes.	Galactose restricted diet and supplemental calcium.
Fructosuria	Fructokinase	Sucrose and honey, and fructose should be avoided.

17. Effect of Age

Patients tend to outgrow their sensitivity to food allergens. Foods known to have caused reactions in childhood may be tried months or years later when perhaps they can be taken with impunity.

Dietary treatment is mainly aimed to eliminate the food which produces allergy. Trial diets including foods known to be allergenic are given to the patient. In such cases exclusion of the allergic food from the dietary is the only effective means to prevent allergy. If infants are born with milk allergy, substitutes must be made through goat's milk or evaporated milk. Soyabean milk may also be used as a substitute since soyabean is very nutritious. Finally, each food that is omitted from the diet should be replaced with one of the similar nutrient value.

18. Nutritional Risk in Food Allergy Management

Level of Risk	Food characteristic / Examples
Low risk	Any food that can easily be eliminated with minimal or no nutritional risk to the patient Example ; Avoidance of a specific fruit or vegetable
Moderate risk	Any food that may be encountered frequently through the food supply, yet whose elimination does not significantly limit food choices or vital nutrient sources Example : Avoidance of fish, crustaceans, and tree nuts.
Complex	Any food that permeates the food supply providing a significant source of specific nutrients that are not readily available through other foods that are a part of the normal diet, whose elimination results in a significant life-style and dietary change owing to the difficulty of avoiding that food an products containing that food. Example : Avoidance of wheat, soy, egg. Milk peanuts, or multiples foods.

19. Strategies for Coping with Food Allergy

i.   Food Substitution

Try to substitute item-to-item at meals. For example if the family is eating icecream for dessert, substitution of another type of frozen dessert may be better accepted than a dissimilar dessert, such as cookies.

ii.   Dining Out and Eating Away from Home

Eating meals away from home can be risky for individuals with food allergies. Whether at a fancy restaurant or a fast-food establishment, inadvertent exposure to an allergen can occur, even among the most knowledgeable individuals. Here are some precautions to take.

- Bring "safe" foods along to make eating out easier. For breakfast bring along soy milk if others will be having cereal with milk.
- Alert the wait staff to the potential severity of your foods allergy
- Question the wait staff carefully about ingredients'
- Always carry medication.

iii.   Special Occasions

Call the host family in advance to determine what foods will be served. Offer to provide an acceptable dish that all can enjoy.

iv.   Grocery Shopping

Be informed about what foods are acceptable and read labels carefully. Product ingredients change over time; continue to read the labels on foods, even if they were previously determined to be "safe" foods. Allows for the fact that shopping will take extra time.

v.   Label Reading

New labeling legislation makes it easier for individuals with food allergies to identify certain potential allergens from the ingredient from the ingredient list on food labels. For example, when food manufacturers use protein hydrolysates or hydrolyzed vegetable protein, they must now specify the source of protein used (e.g., hydrolyzed soy or hydrolyzed cornl. Although reactions to food colors or food dyes are rare, individuals who suspect an intolerance will find them listed separately on the food label. Rather than categorized simply as"Food color".

Substitutions in Cooking

- Milk use soy or rice milk, or fruit juice in recipes calling for milk. Use soy or rice milk for milk replacement, use a 1:1 replacement ratio. Infant formulas, such as neonate, Nutramigen, or Alimentum, can also be used.
- Egg: In baking achieve the emulsifying effect of ne egg by combining 2 T whole wheat flour, ½ tsp oil, ½ tsp baking powder, and 2 T milk, water, or fruit juice. Egg–free substitutes are also available.
- Chocolate: Use carob powder, measure for measure, when substituting for cocoa. As a substitute for one square of chocolate. Use 3 T carob powder plus 2 T milk, water, butter, margarine.
- Wheat: Wheat flour replacements and tips for cooking without wheat are available from many sources.

vi.   *Recommendations for Infant Feeding*

Human milk is the preferred food for all infants. When use of human milk is not possible, soy protein or cow's milk protein hydrolysate formulas are alternatives to standard cow's milk formulas. If symptoms continue, an amino–based formula, may be offered (Hill et al., 1995, Vanderhoof, 1997). Of infants allergic to cow's milk, 15% to 50% may also develop an allergy to soy (Sampson et al., 1991). Use of a protein hydrolysate formula instead of a soy formula in infants who are showing clinical symptoms of an allergic reaction to cow's milk is recommended to reduce the likelihood of sensitization to soy protein also. The American Academy of Pediatrics recommends the use of human milk or casein or whey protein hydrolysaes with peptides having a molecular weight of less than 1200 Daltons for infants with clinical symptoms of cow's milk or soy allergy. Commercially available casein protein hydrolysate formulas (Nutramigen, Pregestimil, and Alimentum) that meet this criterion have routinely been used to feed infants allergic to cow's milk protein, and adverse reactions have only rarely been reported. However, some whey protein hydrolysate formulas (Good Start) contain larger peptides and are not an acceptable alternative for these infants (American Academy of Pediatrics, 1989). The use of goat's milk as an alternative to cow's milk is not recommended because of the potential cross-reactivity with beta–lactoglobulic in cow's milk. In addition, goat's milk is deficient in several nutrients and has a high renal solute load.

It is especially low in folic acid, containing about 1/10 the level present in whole cow's milk or human milk. Infants receiving goat's milk instead of infant receiving cow milk require supplements of iron, folacin, and vitamins A, C, and D. Goat's milk must be diluted to three – quarters strength, and carbohydrates must be added to decrease the renal solute load.

Food Allergy-Checklist

1. There is no guarantee that allergy can be prevented, but there are prophylactic measures that seem well worth taking in the hope of preventing the development of allergy in the allergy–prone new born.

2. If the hypothesis that a fetus may be sensitized in the womb is correct, then a mother to be should eat moderately of a variety of foods during her pregnancy, avoid potently allergenic foods whenever possible and drink no more than a pint of milk daily that has been boiled for ten minutes, if all of this has been approved of by her own doctor.

3. Most important of all, she should do everything possible to ensure that she can breast feed the baby, a measure equally important for the non allergy prone infant as it is for the allergy prone.

4. If the baby is not breast-fed, them under the prophylactic hypothesis he should receive no cow's milk but should have soybean or meat base milk substitute formulas.

5. Eggs should not be introduced until the baby is nine months or a year old and should then be given as hard boiled yolk to begin with.

6. Always begin new foods unmixed with any other food and one single food at a time.

7. Cereals should not be introduced until the baby is at least three months old.

8. Fruits and vegetables may be introduced at four to six months.

9. Meat should wait until the baby is six to nine months old.

10. Diet during an illness and convalescence should be as free of allergenic foods as possible with as little changing about as possible.

11. The allergy prone should avid food fads and an immoderate consumption of a single or a few foods.

12. All of this is relatively uncertain, not wholly proved and not absolute, but it is a better safe than sorry approach to the problem.

13. Each child is an individual and must be treated as such, non allergic and allergy prone alike.

<h1 style="text-align:center">Chapter XI</h1>

<h2 style="text-align:center">Prevention of Food Allergy</h2>

1. Eat a varied Diet, avoid excessive quantities of any one food.
2. Careful reading of commercial food labels should become the way of life for allergic patients.

What causes allergy now may not do so after a few months or a few years. It is therefore wise to abstain from some food stuffs causing allergy and then try again. The type of preparation or form of cooking food stuff may also matter sometimes. For example, some people may be allergic to milk but may tolerate curd or instead of lightly boiled egg may be able to take an egg which has been boiled for at least 10 minutes or tolerate even an omlette.

The identification and treatment of allergies is a complex problem facing the public and the medical profession.

Prevention of Food Allergy

Although it is not a fool proof way to prevent food allergy, delaying the introduction of highly allergenic foods into the diets of infants with a family history of allergy is a wise precaution. The early feeding of solid foods to an infant with an immature gastro intestinal tract in infants invites absorption of an allergen and possible sensitivity. Giving foods such as Wheat, Eggs, Oranges, Chocolate, Fish and Nuts should be postponed. Meats should not be started before 6 to 9 months of age, and lamb and veal, the least allergenic, should be tried first. Breast feeding until this age is also recommended.

Patient Counseling

Many foods contain minute amounts of substances to which some people react. The patient must have detailed lists of foods to use, and foods to avoid.

The meal pattern should fit in with the family's pattern and must be one that assures nutritional adequacy. An allergy to milk means that another source of calcium, usually a calcium supplements must be provided. Soybean substitutes for milk are sometimes fortified with calcium. Allergy to citrus fruits means that other foods that are good sources of ascorbic acid must be emphasized. When there is allergy to wheat it is sometimes necessary to emphasize adequate caloric intake.

A number of recipe booklets are available for patients who are allergic to milk, eggs, or wheat. Rye, corn, rice soy, or potato flours may be used instead of wheat flour. However, they do not contain the gluten in wheat and the textures of products made with these flours are quite different from those to which people are accustomed. Reading labels on food packages and cans and interpreting the information is absolutely essential.

There are two kinds of allergic reaction immediate and delayed. Immediate reactions occural most at once after a person has been exposed to an allergen. Symptoms are apparent within minutes or hours. This type of reaction takes place in the shock organs because, it is thought, these are especially vulnerable to the allergenantibody conflict since the IgEAntibodies are in greater concentrations in these areas. Hay Fever, Asthma, Hives, Sensitivity to insect Bites and Stings and allergy to foods are examples of immediate reaction. Delayed reactions appear hours, days and even weeks after exposure and are caused, it is believed, when antibody – type white blood cells attack allergens so violently that a certain amount of the body's tissue is destroyed. Examples of delayed reaction are allergies to poison ivy. Cosmetic and soaps.

Prognosis

The prognosis for allergy varies with the individual. Some patients are cured, others improved, while still others receive very little aid through treatment. The patient must be impressed with the fact that continuous adherence to the program is necessary to obtain beneficial results. The duration of the treatment depends upon the individual, it may be weeks, months or years.

The patient should have careful, frequent checkups to avoid the unnecessary exclusion of foods and to ingest an adequate diet to correct mistakes, psychosomatic medicine enters into the treatment of allergy, since some patients prefer clinging to symptoms rather than getting well. Others develop the emotional lesion typical in any recurrent disease.

Chapter XII

Conclusion

Allergy is an Allergen(Antigen)-Antibody mediated immunological adverse reaction which is mild, moderate, severe and sometimes fatal due to anaphylactic shock depending on the nature of allergens ingested or inhaled. As a rule of clinical practice, the allergy is so severe in infants and young ones. The severity of allergy is reduced as the age advances as the gastrointestinal system matures and sensitizes person's body immune response. The best way to treat allergy is refrain from causative foods and use of food substitutes. The most common food allergens in young children are Milk, Eggs and Wheat. So the dietary management of allergy is crucial rather than drugs unless situation warrants. This book explains in a crisp manner about the Nature, Symptoms, Treatment and Nutritional Management of Allergy and their prevention and the most important patient counseling. The explanation of allergy in a sequential manner is well understood even for a common man. So the comprehensive review of allergy in this book gives some basic concepts involved in the elicitation of the allergy and their consequences.

Key Terms

Adverse Food Reaction

Any undesired response to a food that is not documented to be allergy based.

Allergen

Substance foreign to the body which, upon interaction with the immune system causes an allergic reaction.

Anaphylaxis

An acute,often severe, and sometimes fatal immune response that may affect one or more organ systems.

Antibodies

Immunoglobulins produced in response to an antigen or allergen.

Atopy

Tendency toward allergies, determined genetically.

Allergen

Any substance capable of producing allergy. Sometimes used interchangeably with antigen.

Allergist

A doctor specializing in the medical subspecialty of allergy.

Allergy

Overreaction to substances normally not harmful to others.

Angioedema

Large, deep swelling; giant hives.

Animal Dander

Skin flakes, scales and scurf.

CAP-RAST FEIA (FLUROSCEIN – ENZYME IMMUNOASSAY): A test, more sensitive than the radioallergosorbent test (RAST), that provide quantitative assessment of food – specific IgE antibodies

Cell Mediated Immunity: Immunity that is mediated by T lymphocytes, either through the release of lymphokines or by direct cytotoxicity.

Cross Reactivity: An allergic response to a food or substance either within a given group (i.e., crustacean, legumes) or with unrelated Substances (e.g., banana, kiwi, or chestnuts with latex)

Dermatitis

Inflammatory condition of the skin.

DOUBLE – BLIND, PLACEBO – CONTROLLED FOOD CHALLENGE (DBPCFC): A test of reaction to a food where the food is disguised such that neither the patient nor researcher knows it is being given; the "gold standard" for establishing food allergy.

Eczema: A skin rash characterized by small red and white bumps that itch; often a symptom of allergy; also called atopic dermatitis.

Edema: A condition in which tissues contain excess fluid; swelling

Elimination Diet: an eating plan that omits one or more foods suspected to cause an adverse food reaction. An eating plan in which individual foods suspected of causing intolerance or allergic reactions are omitted for a period of time in order to determine if there is an improvement in the individual's condition

Food Intolerances

Adversereaction to a normally harmless substance in food that does not involve the body's immune system.An adverse reaction to a food caused by toxic, pharmacologic, metabolic, or idiosyncratic reactions to the food or chemical substances in the food

Food Allergy

Adverse reaction to a normally harmless substance in food that involves the body's immune system. (Also called food Hypersensitivity)

Food and Symptom Diary

A record of food and drink consumed and symptoms experienced

Immune System

Body tissue that provide protection against bacteria, viruses, and other substances identified by cell as harmful.

Humoral Immunity

Immunity mediated by antibodies produced by B lymphocytes Ig E Mediated allergic reaction (Immediate hyper Sensitivity).

IgE antibody–mediated hypersensitivity occurring within minutes after a sensitized individual is exposed to an antigen.

Radio Allergo Sorbent Test (RAST)

A test that measures specific IgE antibodies in serum : used as an alternative to skin tests.

Rotation Diet

An eating plan in which several foods known to cause allergic reactions or which are not tolerated are eaten on separate days and then only every fourth of fifth day for each food.

Sensitization

Exposure to an antigen or allergen that results in the development of hypersensitivity

Skin Test

A test in which an antigen is applied to the skin in order to observe the histamine response of the patient.

Sensitized: Made susceptible to a substance.

Sensitivity

Abnormally susceptible to a substance: used interchangeably with allergy and allergic.any undesired response to a food that is not documented to be allergy based .

References

- Aas K:Antigens in food.Nutr. Rev 42:85,1984.

- Adelle Davis Lat's get well (New York : Harcourt, Brace Jovanovich 1965)

- AllergyRecipiesChicago,II. The American Dietetic Association,1969.

- Allergy : what it is and What To do about it (New York :Ungar 1949, 1966)

- Allergy–Its Mysterious Cause and treatment (New York: Grosset& Dunlap, 1968). Published by Allergy foundation of America

- Allergy–its Treatment and Care .(Toronto, Ontario, Canada; Longmans 1968)

- American Academy of Allergy and Immunology, Committee on adverse Reactions to Foods.NIH Publication No. (NIAID) 84:2442,july 1984.

- American Academy of Pediatrics, Committee on Nutrition: Hypoallergenic infant formulas. Pediatrics 83:1068,1989.

- American Academy of Pediatrics: Hypersensitivity to food. In Forbes GB and Woodruff CW(eds):Pediatric Nutrition Handbook. ElkGroveVillage,IL, American Academy of Pediatrics,1985.

- American Academy of Pediatrics, Committee on Nutrition: Soy protein formulas: Recommendation for use in infant feeding. Pediatrics 72:359. 1983.

- Atkins, F.M: The Basis of Immediate Hypersensitivity Reactions to foods, Nutr.Rev., 41:229-234,1983.

- Atkins FM et al: Evaluation of immediate adverse reactions to food in adult patients.II:A detailed analysis of reaction patterns during oral food challenge.J Allergy ClinImmunol 75:356,1985.

- Bahna S.L. and Gandhi, M.D:MilkHypersensitivity.I. Pathogenesis and Symptomatology, Ann.Allergy, 50:218-223,1983.

- Bahna,s.L.,andGandhi,M.D:MilkHypersensitivity.II. Practical Aspects of Diagnosis, Treatment and Prevention, Ann.Allergy,50:295-301,1983.

- Baking for People with Food Allergies. Home and Garden Bulletin No.147, Washington, D.C. U.S. Department of Agriculture,1976.

- Barbara Yordy Allergy Diet Cookbook (Twin falls, Idaho: Standard printing Company, n.d.)

- Bernhisel-Broadbent J and Sampson H: Cross allergenicity in the legume botanical family in children with food hypersensitivity. Allergy ClinImmunol 83:435,1989.

- Bernstein M, Day JH and Welsh A:Double-blind food challenge the diagnosis of food sensitivity in the adult .J Allergy ClinImmunol 70:205,1982.

- Billie Little Recipes for Allergies (New York : Vantage press 1968)
- Bock SA:A critical evaluation of clinical trials in adverse reactions of foods in children.J. Allergy ClinImmunol 78:165, 1986.
- Bock SA: The natural history of food sensitivity.J Allergy ClinImmunol 69:173,1982.
- BockSA: Natural history of severe reactions to foods in young children. JPediatr 107:676, 1985.
- Bock SA et al: Studies of hypersensitivity reactions to foods in infants and children. J Allergy ClinImmunol 62:327, 1978.
- Bock SA et al:Proper use of skin tests with food extracts in diagnosis of hypersensitivity to food in children. Clin Allergy 7:375, 1977.
- Bush RK et al: Soyabean oil is not allergenic to soybean sensitive individuals. J Allergy ClinImmunol 73:176, 1984.
- Businco L et al: Prevention of atopic diseases in "at risk newborn by prolonged breastfeeding. Ann Allergy 51:296, 1983.
- Businco L et al: Soybean oil is not allergenic to soybean sensities individuals. J Allergy ClinImmunol 51L: 296, 1983.
- Businco, L et al: Prevention of atopy: Results of a long – term Months to 8 Years) follow - upann allergy 59:183, 1987.
- Carol g. Emerling The Allergy Cookbook (Garden city, N.Y: Doubleday 1969)
- Claude A. Frazier Insect Allergy (St.Louis, Mo.: W.H. Green 1969)
- Cole,D:Feeding Allergic Patients,Hospitals,45:95-100,February 16,1971.
- Dannaeus, A: Management of Food Allergy in Infancy, Ann.Allergy, 51:303-306,1983.
- DavidTJ: Unorthodox allergy procedures. Arch Dis Child 62:1066, 1987.
- David TJ, Wacdington E and Stanton RHJ: Nutritional hazards of elimination dietsin children with atopic eczema.ArchDis Childd 59:323, 1984.
- Doris J. Rapp. M.D., Allergies and your child (New York : Holt, Rinehart & Winston 1972)
- Edith Piltz Bland but Grand (Garden City, N.Y. :Doubledary 1970)
- Eggleson PA: Prospective studies in the natural history of food allergy. Ann Allergy 59:179, 1987.
- Egger J et al: Is migraine food allergy? Lancet 2:805, 1983.
- Elizabeth C. Robertson Nutrition for today (Toronto, Ontario Canada: McClelland and stewart Ltd., 1951)

- Environmental Health Association Manual for those sensitive to Foods, Drugs and Chemicals (Washington, D.C., 1969)

- Fomon, Infany Nutrition,2d ed., Saunders Company,Philadelphia,1974,p-414.American Acdemy of Pediatrics, committee on Nutrition: Hypclergenic infant formulas. Pediatrics 83 ; 1068, 1989.

- Felleson,J.A. The clinical ecology unit.RN, 40:49, 1977.

- Florence E. Sammis The Allergic Patient and His world (Springfield, III: C.C. Thoma 1958)

- Frazier, C.A. Coping with Food Allergy, Quadrangle/The New York Times Co.,New York, 1974, p-6.

- Frazier,C.A.(ed.):Current Therapy of Allergy, New York, Medical Examinations Publishing Co.,Inc., 1974, pp.204-223.

- Halpin.T.C..etal:Colitis, Persistent Diarrhoea and Soy Protein Intolerance, J.Pediatr., 91: 404-407,1977.

- Hamburger RN et al: Current status of the clinical and immunological consequences of a prototype allergic disease prevention programmes. Ann Allergy 59:179, 1987.

- Harold W. Bottomly Marion l. Conrad Allergy cooking (New York : T.Y. Crowell 1960.

- Harry F. Swartz The Allergy guide–Book–A practical program of Prevention and control (New York : Unger 1961, 1966)

- Hill DJ et al; Manifestations of milk allergy in infancy; Clinical and immunologic findings. J Pediatr 109:270, 1986.

- Hurwtz, S:AcneVulgaris. Current Concepts of Pathogenesis and Treatment,Am.J.Dis. Child., 133:536-544,1979.

- Jakobasson I and Lindberg T: Cow's milk proteins cause infantile colic in breast – fed infants: A double – blind crossorver study. Pediatrics 71:268, 1983.

- Kidd JM et al: Food dependent exercise induced anaphylaxis.J Allergy ClinImmunol 71: 407, 1983.

- Lawrence RA: Breastfeeding: A Guide for the Medical Profession, 2nded.StLouis,CV Mosby,1985,p 234.

- Loretta .White - The good Egg (New York : Rend McNally 1959)

- MansfieldLEetal: Food allergy and adult migraine: Double-blind and mediator confirmation of allergic etiology. Ann Allergy 55:126, 1985.

- Marshall SG, Bierman CW and Shapiro GG:Otitismedia with effusion in childhood.Ann. Allergy53:370, 1984.

- May, C.D: Food Allergy, In:Fomon.S.J.Infant Nutrition,2nd ed. Philadelphia,W.B.Saunders Co.,1974,pp.435-458.

- McCarthy, E.P. and Frick O.L.: Food Sensitivity: Keys to Diagnosis,J.Pediatr,102:645-652, 1983.

- Minford AMB, MacDonald A and Littlewood JM: Food intolerance and food allergy in children. A review of 68 cases. Arch Dis Child 57:742, 1982.1.Mayer,J: Food Allergies, Postgrad. Med., 47:230-33,june 1970.

- Nilson B. Cooking for special Diets (Baltimore, Md: penguin (No. PH. 95), n.d.)

- Panaush RS: Delayed reactions to foods, food allergy and rheumatic disease. Ann Allergy 56: 500,1986a.

- Parent's Guide to Allergy in Children (Garden City, N.Y: Doubleday, 1973)

- Recipes Containing Goat Products-C.A.V. Barker(Toronto, Ontario, Canada; Coach House Press, (1972)

- Reymond J. Benack What is Allergy? (Springfield, III: G.C. Thomas 1967) Rinkle,H.J.,et al: The diagnosis of food allergy.Arch.Otolaryngol,79:78,1964.

- Rowe A.H: Food Allergy. Its Manifestations and Control and the Elimination Diets. A Compendium, Charles C Thomas,Publishers,Springfield,III.,1972.

- Rowe A.H: Elimination Diets and the Patient's Allergies. Philadelphia, Lea&Febiger, 1984.

- Sampson HA et al: Safety of casein hydrolysate formula in children with cow's milk allergy. J Pediatr 118: 520, 1991.

- Sampson HA:Immunologically-mediated food allergy: The importance of food challenge procedures. Ann Allergy 60:262,1988.

- Sampson HA: Food Allergy.J Allergy ClinImmunol 84(6, pt.2):1062, 1989.

- Schachner L: The Treatment of Acne: A Contempoorary Review, Pediatr.Clin.North Am., 30:501-510.

- Spear K.L. and MullerS.A: Treatment of Cystic Acne with 13-cis-Retinoic Acid, MayoClin.Proc., 58:509-514,1983.

- Speer F, Food Allergy: The 10 Common Offenders, Am.Fam.Physician, 13:106-112, February 1976.

- Taubman B: Parental counseling compared with elimination of cow's milk or soy milk protein for the treatment of infant colic syndrome: A randomized trial. Pediatrics 81:756, 1988.

- Taylor SL et al: Food allergens: Structure and immunologic properties. Ann Allergy 59:93, 1981.
- Tuft L, Allergy Management in Clinical Practise. St.Louis, C.V.Mosby   Co., 1973, pp,132-153.
- Wood M.N, Eating Well on a Wheat Free Diet, Today's Health, 48:60-63, February 1970.
- Woodruff C.W, Milk intolerances. Nutri.Rev., 34:33, 1976.
- Wood Gourmet M.L., F ood on a Wheat free diet (Springfield, Iii: C.C. Thomas 1967)
- Zanjanian M.H, The intestine in allergic diseases.Ann.Allergy, 37:208, 1976.
- Ziegler RS et al; Effect of combined maternal and infant food–allergen avoidance on development of atopy in early infancy: A randomized study. J allergy ClinImmunol 84:72, 1989.